"*Mind, Body, Kitchen* offers a truly holistic approach to health and wellness. Stacey's organized and practical approach helps readers melt away overwhelm in order to finally develop healthy thoughts and healthy habits that last."

—MARIA MARLOWE, The Acne Nutritionist, Creator of the Clear Skin Plan, and Author of *The Real Food Grocery Guide*, and *Be Healthy Everyday*

"Stacey Crew is a compassionate guide on the route toward figuring out what 'a healthier lifestyle' means for you. Full of personal stories, helpful suggestions, and invitations to self-inquiry and reflection, *Mind, Body, Kitchen* is a tool for anyone who's ever felt daunted by making a change. Stacey helps you realize that the change you seek is possible."

—HEIDI BARR, Author of *12 Tiny Things* and Editor of *The Mindful Kitchen*

"*Mind, Body, Kitchen* is thoughtfully written and organized into three parts, 'Creating a Healthy You,' a 'Healthy Kitchen,' and a 'Healthy Home,' with valuable exercises to drive the points home. I learned something from each of the parts which I am eager to implement in my own kitchen, first and foremost the zoning of the kitchen. The mindset reminders to quiet the noise of the world and schedule your self-care are key areas to prioritize. Self-care in the morning helps you win the day. Gratitude and mindset are so important to manifest the life you deserve to live, a life of joy, and feeling good. As a fellow health coach, I know if you don't cook for yourself, you won't feel good, and if you don't feel good, you won't have the energy to live your best life. PS: I'm glad you learned how to cook broccoli!"

—MARIE SCOTT, Functional Medicine Certified Health Coach Speaker, and Author of *Finding Meaning (and Humor) in Widowhood, Firehouses, and Organic Vegetables, 7 Steps to Healing*

"I've read many diet and health books, but Stacey's book takes healthy eating and living to a whole different level. She connects the importance of organization with healthy living. Stacey's gentle step-by-step guidance allowed me to see the 'why' behind my habits. This alone, along with her simple yet valuable tips, have helped me shift and create sustainable healthy habits. Stacey's book will be on the shelf in my home as a reminder of the importance of nurturing myself daily along my wellness journey."

—BONNIE COMPTON, Child and Adolescent Therapist/Parent Coach, Author of *Mothering with Courage*

"As a cookbook connoisseur and a sucker for a great self-help book, I had no idea that there was a book that I've really been waiting for: *Mind, Body, Kitchen*. Neither a recipe collection nor pages of self-talk mantras, this book is truly a guide to help you put your good cooking, lifestyle, and purposeful intentions into practice. Stacey Crew skillfully walks by your side so that you can create pragmatic systems and structures that allow you to live the healthy life you always knew you could live!"

—J. L. FIELDS, Health Coach, Culinary Instructor, and Author of *The Complete Plant-Based Diet, Vegan Baking for Beginners,* and more

"Stacey Crew had me at the title! *Mind, Body, Kitchen*! As a mindfulness coach and the editor of a wellness magazine, I KNOW the importance of embracing a mindset of mind and body. Stacey's addition of 'Kitchen' is brilliant! She takes the reader on a journey of how to use mindfulness and mindset practices to lay a solid foundation on which to build a healthy body. She then adds in easy techniques and inspiring motivation to bring more movement into our lives. Finally, by adding the bonus of kitchen organization, she gives her readers everything they need to successfully transform their lives to live healthier and happier! This book is a must-read for those who want to kick the word 'diet' out of their lives and invite in a full transformation to healthy living! In today's fast-paced and chaotic world, Stacey Crew brings a breath of fresh air and a pinch of organization with her book *Mind, Body, Kitchen: Transform You and Your Kitchen for a Healthier Lifestyle*. Filled with personal stories, interesting anecdotes, and practical information, it assists you in creating small changes in your life and kitchen that will truly be a game changer in not only your life but also your health."

—DR STEPHANIE ZGRAGGEN, DC, MS, CNS, CCN, Natural Female Hormone Expert

"The fact that our food, kitchen, and even our cooking utensils can make us ill is a powerful motivator for healthier living. *Mind, Body, Kitchen* takes us on a freshening journey through the best approaches for reducing toxic chemicals in our lives, while inspiring long-lasting lifestyle changes for optimal health."

—ALY COHEN, MD, Integrative Rheumatologist, Best-Selling Author of *Non-Toxic: Guide to Living Healthy in a Chemical World*, and Founder of TheSmartHuman.com

"Crews' approach is holistic; she gently coaches readers to make small, steady changes. By adopting a basic, commonsense approach to nourishing our minds and bodies, we learn how to do better and be better, save money, cook healthy meals at home, and streamline kitchen clutter. Packed with plenty of delicious little reminders for becoming the best version of ourselves."

—GERALIN THOMAS, Author of *From Hoarding to Hope: Understanding People Who Hoard and How to Help Them*

"Stacey Crew eloquently integrates the three pillars of well-being in her book *Mind, Body, Kitchen*. A powerful read that allows us to dive into the how-to of health, from clearing out the toxins in our home and body to informative tips and ideas for reducing stress. Stacey's expertise with organization and nutrition is the perfect backdrop to bring forward all her knowledge that helps each of us be the healthiest we can be. Thank you, Stacey, for putting this all into one book so we just don't visualize health but have clear, concise steps to get there!"

—LUCIE DICKENSON, Author of *Overreacting: A Memoir of Anxious Proportions*

"Stacey's book is chock-full of useful and practical information that goes a long way in making sustainable life changes."

—L. B. ADAMS, CEO and Conversation Catalyst, Practical Dramatics

"If you're looking to transform your life in an organized and healthy manner, Stacey's book is for you. Stacey not only thoughtfully lays out a plan for you to organize your kitchen and home but also gives reasons why. Throughout the book are personal anecdotes from Stacey and client examples illustrating how an organized life is actually simpler to maintain than most of us realize. She clearly outlines steps you need to take without overwhelm. As a health coach, Stacey is deeply committed to guiding clients to live their best life. Her book is no different. This book is for everyone!"

—DEBRA NEGRIN, INHC, SELF Integrative Health

"As someone who faced and overcame a major illness at age forty, I live by the mantra that health is wealth. Stacey is a true inspiration and expert for those looking to increase their overall health and wellness IQ and learn how to integrate mind, body, and nutrition for optimum wellness and vitality. This book provides a wealth of information in a way that is simple and clear to understand and implement day to day. I am excited to share this book with family and friends."

—KELLY GEORGE, Founder, Still Soul Studio

"*Mind, Body, Kitchen* is an informational guide full of helpful tips for living your healthiest life. Whether your focus is on physical health or mental health, Crew makes it easy to start or continue your journey to a healthy and intentional you."

—SHEILA HILL, Founder of Lifestyle Blog piecesofamom.com

"Stacey understands that healthy eating encompasses more than the food that you put in your mouth. She addresses your mindset, routine, and space as well as your nutrition as parts of a whole to help you succeed. Her recommendations and practices work together like a well-oiled machine to help your body run optimally from top to toes."

—CHRISTY LINGO, Professional Organizer, Owner of Simple Solutions Organizing, and Podcast Host of *Cocktails and Containers*

"Stacey really takes the time with her reader to lay out the fundamentals needed to make long-lasting change. Change isn't easy; it takes work, but Stacey uses her knowledge, experiences, and wit to show the reader how it can be done. *Mind, Body, Kitchen* is a wonderful gift for those looking to up-level their life."

—KATHLEEN OSWALT, Registered Dietitian, eatloveTRIATHLON

"I love that *Mind, Body, Kitchen* takes into consideration that change happens—by looking at the whole picture, not just trying tactical strategies. As an organizer, I try to work with this principle with my clients every day! I even saw myself in this book, as I realized that I'm the kind of person who buys fresh produce hoping that I will be inspired to make something out of it, often only to ignore it and eventually compost it. It isn't just about buying good ingredients; it's about how it fits into the full picture."

—KATHY VINES, CPO®, Clever Girl Organizing®

"Thank you, Stacey, for writing this book! It wonderfully captures the connection between organization and living a healthy lifestyle. I love the ideas she proposes in this book, including 'going back in time' to the original purpose of the fridge and being intentional about the stuff we choose to keep in our kitchen. Stacey gives practical advice that's fun and easy to read. If you're a busy person, this book covers a lot of great info in a short amount of time. Any family would sincerely benefit from implementing these strategies in their home."

—JEN VAN BUSKIRK, Family Organization Coach, Neat Mama

"Stacey Crew has just the right combination of skills and experience to take you by the virtual hand and help you overcome the daily obstacles and lead you one step at a time to a calmer, more nutritious, and more fulfilling life. I'm all about clever shortcuts, and I love this book's tips for supercharging your health with easy, doable steps, and minimizing the excess in your kitchen and in your mind. With its interactive journal format, this book will become your own unique guide to better living."

—AVIVA GOLDFARB, Founder of the Six O'Clock Scramble, and Food Marketing and PR Expert

"Stacey Crew has done it! Integrated our knowledge about what to eat and how to get exercise in our lives with mindful planning for everything from shopping to working out. Reading and following her advice in *Mind, Body, Kitchen* will make you feel healthier and happier!"

—HOWARD PRAGER, Author of *Make Someone's Day: Becoming a Memorable Leader in Work and Life*

"In my work as a business coach, I often remind my clients of the importance of taking care of themselves first. It's like they tell you on the airplane: 'Put on your oxygen mask first before helping others.' It doesn't always feel natural to do so, but if we want to show up fully and truly serve others, we must be at our best. I love Stacey's approach to caring for our mind and body first, because this is how we truly set ourselves up to win."

—**HILARY JOHNSON, Business Coach, Founder of Hatch Tribe**

"Stacey has a special ability to help others understand that transforming your space can lead to healthier habits to reach your goals."

—**VALERIE SKINNER, Personal Chef, Blogger, thymeandjoy.com**

"This book has been a lifesaver and a health home run. The beauty of Stacey is her ability to take the overwhelm out of living your best life. So often we get caught up in thinking we can't possibly take on the tasks required to have ultimate vitality, but Stacey provides a clear path to give your body and mind the care it deserves. From helping readers understand the importance of nutrition to walking through strategies and sharing best practices, this book provides the road map you need to exceed your health and wellness goals. As a business owner and busy mother of two young children, it's been a game changer for my family."

—**WHITNEY MCDUFF, Speaker Brand Strategist, PR, Author**

"As a busy mother of three and an entrepreneur, I know how hard it can be to prioritize your health and wellness amid the busyness of daily life. I also know how crucial it is to focus on creating healthy habits. I love how Stacey Crew's book *Mind, Body, Kitchen: Transform You and Your Kitchen For a Healthier Lifestyle*, with its actionable steps and practical information, helps you transform yourself and your environment so you can prioritize a 'body first, business second' mindset that is so important to success, both at home and at work."

—**HELENA ALKHAS, Professional Organizer, Speaker, Author**

"Stacey puts all the pieces of the puzzle together to take back control of these three essential areas in your life—mind, body, and kitchen—and she does it an easy-to-follow format, walking you through each part step-by-step. The book is packed with practical tips and tricks that anyone can try that come from her personal experience as a health coach, but also from her own journey to a healthier lifestyle. She is such an inspiring, heartfelt coach and cheerleader, I can't think of anyone else that I would want by my side on my own journey to a more fulfilling and rewarding life."

—DANIELLE WECKSLER, Professional Recipe Developer, Personal Chef

Mind, Body, Kitchen:
Transform You and Your Kitchen
for a Healthier Lifestyle

by Stacey Crew

© Copyright 2021 Stacey Crew

ISBN 978-1-64663-450-7

Published by

◤ köehlerbooks ™

3705 Shore Drive
Virginia Beach, VA 23455
800-435-4811
www.koehlerbooks.com

mind, body, kitchen

TRANSFORM YOU AND YOUR KITCHEN
FOR A HEALTHIER LIFESTYLE

STACEY CREW

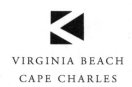

VIRGINIA BEACH
CAPE CHARLES

Dedicated to Claire & Jen and everyone who is attempting to create a healthier lifestyle.

Disclaimer

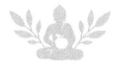

THE INFORMATION SHARED IN this book is for educational and informational purposes only and is not intended to be viewed as medical or mental health advice. It is not designed to be a substitute for professional advice from your physician, therapist, attorney, accountant, or any other health care practitioner or licensed professional. The Publisher and the Author do not make any guarantees as to the effectiveness of any of the techniques, suggestions, tips, ideas, or strategies shared in this book as each situation differs. The Publisher and Author shall neither have liability nor responsibility with respect to any direct or indirect loss or damage caused or alleged by the information shared in this book related to your health, life, or business, or any other aspect of your situation. It's your responsibility to do your own due diligence and use your own judgment when applying any techniques or situations mentioned in or through this book.

Table of Contents

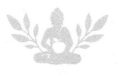

• *Part Three: Creating a Healthy Home* •

Introduction

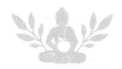

ARE YOU ONE OF the many who has become tired of the ups and downs of dieting, wondering why you can't keep the weight off and what's wrong with you?

Well, let me first tell you that there's NOTHING wrong with you. Secondly, you don't need to diet—because diet implies restrictions.

What you may need to do is shift your mindset, move your body a little more, and learn how to make healthier choices to create a sustainable, healthier lifestyle.

Since my early twenties, I've been exploring and applying self-improvement modalities, using everything from books to seminars to therapy to group counseling to podcasts and online training courses. Now, at mid-life—after marrying, buying and selling homes, having two children, divorcing, and raising two daughters—I understand that learning and change is a lifelong process; it's truly the small, daily shifts that result in big changes over time. In fact, the learning process involves a lot of trial and error, mistakes, setbacks, and failures. Not surprisingly, the failures are where we learn the most.

As a professional organizer for many years, I helped people declutter and organize their homes, which was gratifying. However, I knew something was missing. That is when I began to see that in order to make a space truly functional and healthful, I first had to scrutinize what I was actually organizing. This was especially true in the kitchen.

This book was born after I started making some bigger changes in my life, which included becoming a Certified Health and Wellness Coach after running an organizing business for more than twelve years. Health is a holistic game; the missing ingredients for true health include mindset, nutrition, and movement.

In this book, I've combined what I see as the three pillars of health into a Mind Body Kitchen approach to a healthier lifestyle. Having this realization led me to create a system for myself—and now for you—that addresses MIND, BODY, AND KITCHEN. Let me explain:

MIND: In order to make change—long-lasting, permanent change—one must get their thinking right. If we continue entertaining the same thoughts, we will not move the needle, no matter how hard we try.

> *"We can't solve problems by using the same kind of thinking we used when we created them."*
> —ALBERT EINSTEIN

People try hard all the time. Look at the hundreds of diets introduced that exist and we still have a huge weight issue in this country. Most diets simply focus on the food and neglect a critical part of what needs to happen to change behaviors and habits: mindset. Also, a diet that's right for one person isn't necessarily right for another. And my BIG question: what do you eat when the diet is over?

This book includes the basics of nutrition that empower you to make positive choices, but we start by creating a solid foundation—a shift in mindset—which is the key to permanent change.

BODY: Without some form of movement in our lives and feeding the body healthy foods, we can't effectively make the changes in our body that we'd like to see.

> *"Exercise should be regarded as a tribute to the heart."*
> —GENE TUNNEY

As with our thinking, movement and nutrition must occur in order to create the sustainable change we are seeking. And it's ONLY the combination of the two that will result in the permanent change.

As you'll see in Chapter 3, you simply want to find what works for you and feels right for your body and where you are in your life. Creating a simple routine, even if it means dancing in the kitchen while making dinner, can lift your mood and help you move throughout the day more easily.

KITCHEN: We are more empowered when we know what we're eating, and one of the key ways to do this is to prepare food ourselves.

People are happier *when their kitchen is full of healthy ingredients and they can easily prepare simple, healthy meals.*

This book provides you with simple steps to create a healthy and organized kitchen so you can easily meal plan, shop, and prepare food—and always have something healthy on hand to nourish your body. This section of the book also provides you with the tools needed to organize your kitchen in a way that's efficient, making the process of getting in and out of the kitchen simple and easy.

The Mind Body Kitchen approach will save you time and help you get on the road to a healthier lifestyle in a way that is straightforward and easy to understand. I've taken what I've learned over the years and condensed it into bite-sized pieces of information and processes. You may not find any brilliant or cutting-edge information in this book, but what you will find is that the information is organized in a way that will shortcut your road to healthier eating.

The overall purpose of this book is to provide you with the shortcuts to creating a simple, healthy "diet" and a lifestyle that helps you feel more energized and better at any age. I feel better in my fifties than I did in my thirties, and it's largely due to eliminating processed foods and adding more movement to my daily routine. But the biggest change has been my mindset and the ability to demonstrate a level of self-compassion that I didn't know existed. Without these changes, I would not be writing this book today.

The timing is right too because so many beautiful writers have paved the way by introducing terms and concepts such as self-care, self-compassion, grace, and courage, which makes it easier for me to communicate my ideas without diving deep into what those topics mean. The context has already been established. If you do want to take a deeper drive into these topics, I've included a list of books in the Resource section.

Imagine if you could make the time to discover what you need to do to gain more control over your personal health and wellness, then create a plan to regain control in your life. A simple yet effective system that takes you from feeling lethargic, sluggish, and stressed to energetic, hopeful, and successful. Imagine eliminating what no longer serves you and filling your life with only what fills you up and nourishes your soul.

You're in the right place. Today is your day to get started on a healthier version of you, as well as creating a healthier heart of the home—in the kitchen.

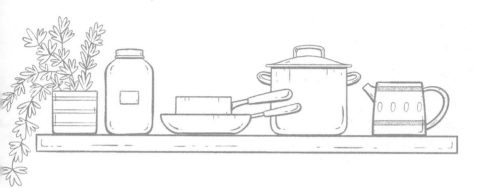

Part One

CREATING A HEALTHY YOU

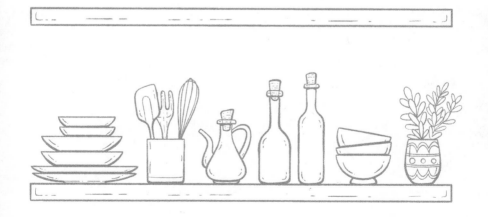

CHAPTER 1

Discovering You

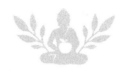

FOR MANY YEARS, I was determined to keep up with the Joneses. I longed to have the newest model of a car, wear the latest clothing trends, and acquire the latest and greatest stuff. I focused on external appearances and not on what fed my soul or filled me with joy.

What I thought was the pursuit of happiness actually threw me into a state of anxiety and left me constantly wondering what came next. I was on the proverbial hamster wheel, and it was only getting faster and faster.

In January 2012, my anxiety was at an all-time high. I wasn't moving my body regularly. I had also adopted some habits that included too much caffeine, not enough self-care, and a penchant for crappy TV.

After a lot of back and forth in my head about what steps I should take, I decided to go to the gym. I'm telling you this story because although this may not be your answer, it was mine and it helped. Maybe this story will inspire you to find your solution. This story also leads into how the Mind Body Kitchen approach began to take shape.

It had been years since I showed up at a workout facility, but my racing thoughts and gnawing sense of restlessness had to go. I told myself that all I just needed to commit to thirty minutes on the treadmill. Once on the treadmill, I walked, then I ran, then I almost heaved because I felt so awful, so I went back to walking, and then I ran again. I stayed on the treadmill for thirty minutes and when I got off, I felt exhausted, but accomplished. So much so that I went back again and again. Three months later, I ran a 10K. Ten months after that I finished a half marathon.

Fitness led me to look more closely at my life. I took inventory of the people I was surrounding myself with and my attitude toward self-care. Then I began to make some pretty big changes. Four years later, I became a certified health and wellness coach helping people improve their diet and lifestyle.

But like you, I'm living in a busy world where so much is expected of us each day. We care for our family, our home, our career and all the things that come with being an adult. And then we experienced the unexpected life-changing situation of the pandemic.

Even as we slowed down during 2020, many people had to step up even more, working from home while homeschooling the kids. This relegated any form of self-care to the bottom of the list and left so many of us feeling overwhelmed and downright burned out.

If we're not careful and don't take control of what we can as we emerge from what we hope is a once-in-a-lifetime event, we can quickly return to letting other people's expectations dictate our lives. The stuff and time commitments will continue to require us to earn more money to pay for what we accumulate, or intend to accumulate. Then managing the stuff potentially becomes almost a full-time job.

The time constraints have us zipping through the drive-through, telling ourselves that we won't do it again, that it was just because TODAY there wasn't enough time to shop, prepare, and cook healthy meals. Then it happens again, and again, becoming an unstoppable habit that's hard to break.

Stress builds and we become anxious. Once this happens, our mental and physical health begins to suffer. We can experience self-doubt, confusion, and physical symptoms such as headaches, stomach issues, or skin irritations. But we're not sure why because "everyone" tells us this is what we're supposed to want and we're slowly discovering that keeping up is not making us happy. We're left stressed and worn out.

When we become more and more entrenched in the satisfaction of external pursuits, the result is a life in which we no longer honor what we truly need and want. Since influences are everywhere, it's critical to determine what's most important to us.

When we're younger, our body and mind can withstand a little neglect with fewer consequences. But as we grow older, physical symptoms can creep in and we wind up with things like anxiety, skin irritations, stomach disorders, and more—all because we haven't taken the time to consider if what we're currently doing even still works. And once we show symptoms, this usually involves a trip to the doctor who is trained to diagnose and prescribe medication based on symptoms, which can start another cycle.

Finding the time to make change can be challenging. It typically means learning to say "no," potentially cutting back on work hours, and incorporating new routines that include exercise and a change in eating habits.

Sarah's Story

Sarah came to me because she wanted to lose weight, which is a common health goal—especially for women. That is often the barometer for how "well" a woman is doing—the number on the scale—which is a sorely mistaken notion. There are many other ways to measure success that include energy levels, sleep patterns, and overall mood.

Back to Sarah. During our initial session, Sarah revealed that she had three children ages fifteen, twelve, and one; a husband; a dog; and a full-time job. She had numerous health issues and concerns, some of which stemmed from recently discovering her birth parents' health issues. The new information was a huge emotional weight that was holding Sarah back because she fully processed the information.

Sarah also admitted she didn't take time for self-care. With three kids, one of whom was still a baby, she felt overwhelmed with the daily grind and regularly put her needs at the bottom of her list, allowing others to do the same by not speaking up and communicating.

To help Sarah, we first determined the best day and time each week to shop for groceries and how to prepare meals in advance, including breakfast, lunch, and dinner. This would save her time before and after work each day. She also enlisted the help and support of her husband. He too worked long hours but had flexibility in his schedule to pick up their one-year-old from daycare each afternoon. Sarah committed to walking the neighborhood at least three times a week in the evening for fifteen minutes by putting the baby in the stroller and inviting her family to come along, but her walk was not dependent upon whether they joined.

By making these small shifts, Sarah and her family created solid habits that allowed her to incorporate additional changes, such as a weekly yoga class on Saturday mornings.

Carving out time for self-care in our schedules can be challenging. And if you're a parent, you're challenged even more to find creative ways to make time for you because somebody will always need something. But as the expression goes, "If mama ain't happy, then nobody's happy."

That's why it's important to review weekly schedules and time-block activities that require you to be at a certain place at a certain time. This includes work and school, scheduled lessons or gym classes for you or the kids, counseling sessions or a church group, among others. Once you've time-blocked those activities, begin to build in scheduled times for meal planning, grocery shopping, meal preparation, and self-care practices (i.e. reading a book, taking a walk, etc.).

Well-meaning family and friends will continue to push their agenda on you, potentially derailing your good efforts and zapping your energy to the point where you give in and fall back on habits that no longer serve you or give you the results you seek. That's why it's critical to consult with yourself on what is right for you.

The noise of the world will also continue. Weeding through all the options can stop you in your tracks before you've even taken your first step. By mid-life, we begin to realize that the introduction of new fads happen regularly and it's just a matter of time before spinning and barre or Paleo are replaced by yet another fabulous creation. Collect only so much information, then decide for yourself, because in the end it's up to you to turn the noise off, assess your personal situation, and make decisions that are based on your personal needs.

SMALL STEPS EQUAL BIG RESULTS

To create change, consistent effort in a forward direction is essential. And doing something is better than nothing. Try not to get stuck in decision fatigue, which we'll discuss later in the book. Failing to establish a plan of action can mean the difference between success and failure. I don't know about you, but failure doesn't feel good—repeated failure can also have negative effects on our self-esteem, so make a plan!

Let's equate not having a health plan to a poorly-thought out house renovation, which can make the project take longer and require more money than initially considered. Worse, you don't get the results you wanted or expected.

Say you decide to upgrade the kitchen and you get hyper-focused on the flooring without looking at the bigger picture—in this case, the rooms that are adjacent to the kitchen. You measure, buy, and install the flooring only in the immediate area. When you look at the finished flooring afterwards, you see how the flooring in the dining room is obviously different, and now you're frustrated. Then you realize if you had just thought a little bigger, you could've replaced the dining room floor too for just a few hundred dollars more. Instead, you're left kicking yourself that you rushed the project and how you'll likely need to upgrade the dining room floor when you put the house on the market in order to compete with other properties in the neighborhood.

Health is similar because you can hyper-focus on one area without considering the overall picture of your health. For example, weight. You want to lose weight so you quickly make a decision to join a gym for hundreds of dollars a year, then realize there's not enough money in the budget to address the nutritional needs required to really push your health goals forward. In this case, it may have made more sense to spend hundreds of dollars on working with a nutritionist or health coach, with a few personal training sessions, to clearly identify how to reach your ultimate goals.

We've all made quick decisions when we want to make change. Hey, I joined a gym on the same day I decided I no longer wanted to experience anxiety (thankfully it just cost ten dollars a month.) So, if you've made one of these impulsive decisions, don't worry. This book is here to help guide you to make informed decisions based on your personal needs that fit into both your schedule and budget.

To wrap up this chapter, I want you to imagine it's one year from now and your life will be exactly the same as it is today . . .

Would you be okay with that? How would that make you feel?

_____

_____

_____

_____

If nothing changes, what are the consequences to your self-esteem, your health, your family and friends, your lifestyle, and career?

_____

_____

_____

_____

_____

How important is it to overcome these personal challenges in your life?

_____

_____

_____

_____

_____

In the next chapter, you'll create a solid foundation to move forward. Without this, any attempts to improve your health will be shaky at best. So let's make sure your thinking is clear, you're facing the reality of your current situation, and you're focused on the future and your goals.

CHAPTER 2

Foundation

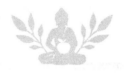

A STRONG FOUNDATION IS necessary for long-term, permanent change.

I love to define words to make sure we're using them correctly. It's also important for us to be on the same page. So, for the purposes of this chapter, let's begin by defining the word *foundation*.

Webster's Dictionary defines foundation as "an underlying basis or principle for something." In terms of a house, the foundation is what holds up the entire structure. Or in a relationship, the foundation is made of core values. When it comes to health and wellness, my definition of foundation is the knowledge to make informed decisions that will benefit your health.

When we begin to create a foundation, inevitably a transformation —a "thorough or dramatic change in form or appearance"—occurs.

All of this takes commitment—a commitment to feeling uncomfortable and awkward because any time we attempt to make change, it can get a little messy before the change even occurs. I'm sure you have a story or two about how if you just stuck with something for a little longer, you would've seen different results. I've got a few of those stories, too!

One way to understand the transformational process is to remember the learning curve when starting a new job. There's the period of learning and working through expectations, there's meeting new co-workers and learning how to collaborate with them, and there's the extra time and effort it takes in order to get comfortable with new processes and procedures. Then, one day, it all magically clicks and you're comfortable. You know what you're doing and you're even surpassing your own expectations.

Adopting new lifestyle changes and behaviors works the same way. There's a learning curve, which means there will be some discomfort, adjustments, and finally the moment when things begin to click. But it all takes time.

And as with a job, once you've gained confidence and mastered your role, you'll likely consider applying for a promotion, moving to a new company, or maybe even starting your own business. Whatever decision you make, you will again begin the cycle. The health game is no different. You incorporate change, you put in the extra time, and then one day it's like magic and you're feeling confident and seeing results. And then you're ready to take it to the next level, which will involve a little discomfort, but you begin to accept that it's all part of the process.

Megan's Story

For years, Megan would make progress with her health goals, then become derailed or distracted by other things in her life, including a new job opportunity and other people's needs. She wanted so badly to succeed at a healthier lifestyle but couldn't stay focused long enough on herself. These attempts eluded her for most of her adult life.

Distractions included the many family and friends she loved dearly but who always seemed to need or want something from her. This prevented her from creating the time she needed to exercise regularly and eat healthier. Granted, she could've said no, but that wasn't part of her family culture or friend circle. People would show up unexpectedly or text her to see what she was doing and the next thing Megan knew, she was out the door going to the latest restaurant or one of the many events in her town or a newly-opened boutique.

What Megan really craved was connection, which she got through these interactions, but at the same time, they drained her because she was spending money she didn't have buying things that she really didn't need and eating foods that didn't contribute to a healthier lifestyle.

After many years, this began to take a toll on her physical and emotional health, as well as her financial situation.

When Megan came to see me, she felt stressed, and she wanted to lose some weight. She felt she was drinking too much wine, and we discovered she was not eating enough nutritious foods to allow her body to thrive.

Megan had tried many diets, most of which she white-knuckled her way through because she did it only because she thought she *should*, not because she felt motivated or inspired to create healthy habits. She had ideas about how she wanted to feel, but she didn't actually want to put in the effort to get to the other side—meaning addressing the emotions and reasons she allowed the distractions to continue. Anytime these uncomfortable emotions surfaced, she would text a friend or get in the car to go see the very people who were also struggling with making positive changes. Ultimately, they proverbially threw their hands up and went to brunch or went shopping, avoiding the necessary work. We've all been there!

Oftentimes, we don't hang in there long enough to see the results. We don't understand that it takes daily, consistent effort over a period of time to make change. We give up after a week because we get uncomfortable and don't want to experience the emotions that come up during the period of change. We quit before the magic happens.

With Megan, we began with small shifts. After our first session, she agreed to give herself what we called "Five Days of Freedom." This meant that she would alert her family and friends that she was trying something new, and she asked them for space to acclimate. If they pushed for details, she would simply tell them she was attempting to make dietary changes and would be eating at home for the next five nights. She knew they would joke and express sarcasm because that's what they'd always done, but Megan agreed to stick to the plan.

This was a big shift for Megan because she had never been completely loyal to herself when it came to change. She would always check in with the people who didn't provide any real support, people who would joke and throw out a lot of unsupportive banter. Now that Megan was aware of this, she was off to a good start.

We met every other week, but Megan found that a daily check-in with someone supportive was also helpful. She identified a friend from work who was a great fit for this role because she had been living a healthy and active lifestyle as long as Megan had known her. Megan trusted her, and the woman agreed to help. Megan would check in with her face-to-face at work and in the evening with a text.

Through our continued coaching sessions, Megan opened up about her beliefs and we uncovered the root of why she hadn't maintained change over the years: Megan knew her parents loved her very much, but they always expected her to strongly abide by their rules and what they told her to do. She'd become "agreeable" in order to get along and stay in good standing with her parents. This followed her into adulthood, not only continuing with her parents, but with other people, too. By the time she reached thirty, she was well into people-pleasing mode and living up to everyone's expectations. She was someone you could count on for almost anything at the drop of a hat, to the detriment of herself.

This discovery changed everything for Megan. It helped her to understand why she often over-indulged with food and wine, which had become a coping mechanism. Instead of facing how she felt head-on, she would drink, eat, and shop.

We began by making small changes in how she responded to others. She did two things: first, she turned the ringer on her phone off and, second, she agreed to always place the phone face down when it wasn't in her hand. Her phone had constantly beeped and buzzed, each time triggering a surge of cortisol through her body because she suspected someone wanted something from her.

She didn't want to go cold turkey and cut people off completely, but instead she learned how to set healthy boundaries. Turning off the ringer and only checking her phone once an hour was a good compromise that created some space so she could breathe. This allowed her to have quiet time and listen to her gut and intuition. Megan also had an opportunity to get her thoughts together before returning a call or text message.

With food, we started her off with my Three-Day Jumpstart (located in the back of this book). Megan began preparing meals and snacks to take to work for lunch, allowing her to eat healthier while saving money. She was creating a solid foundation!

• Creating a Daily Routine •

Starting the day off on the right foot is part of creating and maintaining a solid foundation for self-care and going out into the world. When we jump out of bed and rush through getting ready without stopping to take time to set the tone, we may never feel fully prepared, present, or mindful during the day.

There are several practices that can set a positive tone for the day. Here are a few suggestions; choose one or all and incorporate others as they work for you. If you already feel rushed in the morning, consider waking up a little earlier. If you're someone who hits the snooze button a couple of times before getting out of bed, you may want to schedule a routine for later in the day. And if you have kids and the day starts off like a relay race, then maybe you find time in the evening after they've gone to sleep.

Connecting with yourself is the goal, so do it when it works best for you. This is not something to simply check off your to-do list. So whether it's a five-minute meditation, a quick tally in your mind of what you're grateful for, or a full-on thirty- to sixty-minute practice, find a way to make time for the most important person in your world—you!

MEDITATION

Meditation is something I learned and have practiced on and off for many years, but I began to embrace it more fully when I started practicing yoga in 2015. Meditation offers a focused period of attention on nothing but your breathing. Granted, it's not easy, especially if you're Type-A with lots of things to get done. But as I heard a few of my yoga teachers say from time to time, yoga is a "practice," not a "perfect."

Meditation is also a great way to regain balance and calm, a way to understand yourself and even find answers. I saw a funny meme once that said, "Meditation: because some questions can't be answered by Google." True. Google doesn't know how I feel and it can't replicate one's inner wisdom—not yet, anyway.

Creating space each day for meditation can help us tap into a resource that's available to us anytime—our gut, which is also considered the second brain. This can mean that if the gut is literally clogged with gunk from bad food, our intuition isn't available to us either, so that's another important reason to clean up one's diet and regain full access to inner wisdom.

Just as important as drinking lots of water or eating greens each day, meditation offers us a valuable instrument in our foundational toolbox. The practice can be as simple as setting a timer on our phone for five minutes while sitting in quiet surroundings with our eyes closed. Or not. Some people are able to access "quiet" in the midst of chaos, too. That's the dream.

A simple way to begin to embrace meditation is to sit comfortably, put your feet on the floor, place your palms face-up on your lap, close your eyes, and breathe slowly and steadily, in through your nose and out through your mouth. Long, slow breaths. When thoughts come to mind, dismiss them by mentally by swiping right—or left—your choice. Don't worry, plenty more will come.

We experience about 60,000 thoughts per day, most of which go unrecognized. It's the ones we latch onto and entertain that can become internalized beliefs if we think those thoughts long enough. A belief is simply a thought repeated over and over again.

Meditation offers a way to gain an understanding of what's happening in our bodies and mind through quieting the mind and noticing the breath.

After you've completed the simple instructions above, sweep your arms up and over your head and bring them into a prayer position at your heart, if you choose. I try to end with a smile and a thought of gratitude as a way to acknowledge that I've done something positive for myself and created space in the day to check in with what's happening internally.

There are lots of apps (see the Resources section), YouTube videos, meditation studios, and even retreats to help you get started and learn what works for you. The overall goal is to quiet your mind and find some peace.

GRATITUDE

How often do we complain about things only to one day realize complaining has just become a bad habit? One of my all-time favorite spiritual gurus is Wayne Dyer. He would always say, "When you change the way you look at things, the things you look at change." Gratitude can help us get there and adjust our mindset so we go from feeling that it's impossible to feeling that it's possible. This is the off-ramp of complaining.

Gratitude, by nature, has a positive effect on both the mind and body. When we think about what we're grateful for and summon emotions associated with those positive thoughts, the brain releases natural chemicals—dopamine and serotonin—that enhance our mood and make us feel good. I'm not telling you anything scientifically new here, of course. Just pointing out that it is within our control to feel good—gratitude is the conduit that allows us to feel good in a safe and healthy manner—anytime you want!

Many believe that when we focus on the positive, or the good, the universe delivers more of it. I believe that. So much so that I kept a gratitude book for our family when my children were little. Every night before we read books at bedtime, we would ask each other what we were grateful for and write the answers in a red, leather-bound book I still have today. Some of my daughter's answers sounded downright silly to me, but it always made us smile and developed into something that they still practice today. Starting the day off with a short gratitude list—whether written or just acknowledged in your mind—can truly set the tone for the entire day.

INSPIRATIONAL READING

Another way to set the stage for the day and create a solid foundation is to read something inspirational: either a couple of pages from a favorite book or an entire chapter of a book you're working through.

This inputs something positive into your mind or, at the very least, provides ideas that you can come back to throughout the day. This type of reading can also create inspiration and focus for the day ahead. Instead of being frustrated by the morning commute, you can reflect on what you've read. This may also give you fodder for lunchtime conversation and an avenue to connect with coworkers or help solve a problem.

Inspirational reading is also a good morning practice if you journal and are looking for a prompt to begin writing.

JOURNALING

As I've mentioned, health is much more than just the food we eat and the exercise we accomplish. A healthy mind is critical to sustainable, long-lasting change. As Albert Einstein said, "We cannot solve our problems with the same thinking we used when we created them."

Journaling is helpful in this respect because it allows us to process feelings and express emotions that we otherwise may not communicate verbally. We can sort through feelings of frustration, anger, resentment, confusion, and even jealousy. It's a private space where we can be honest, unfiltered, uncensored, and completely transparent to gain clarity and perspective on a situation.

It's also a place for creative thought. You may consider drawing pictures to represent feelings and emotions. Also, when we return to previously written journal entries, we can notice the experience of transformation and healing that builds strength and self-confidence. Your journal can also be a place where you write your gratitude list, expressing the joy and growth you see in your everyday life.

ADDITIONAL FOUNDATION TOOLS

You can also create change in the following ways:

1. **Put yourself in the driver's seat.** Understand and embrace the idea that this is your life. You're the creator and director of your movie. No one else! Therefore, when it comes to deciding what you want your life to look like, you only need to consider yourself in that moment. This doesn't mean make immediate and drastic changes or dismiss the people closest to you. But it does mean considering how you want to feel and where you want to be ultimately. Stop being the passenger. Take the wheel and figure out what you love and what no longer serves you. Make a list and begin to eliminate what's no longer needed so you can then embrace what you love and what will get you to your ultimate goal.

2. **Make conscious decisions.** No more random decisions.
    Remove the auto-pilot setting, look at what you're doing
    each day and see what doesn't fit with the bigger picture.
    If ultimately you want to be healthy and fit, but you're
    drinking beer every weekend, that may not be the best
    decision. If you want to be emotionally free, yet you're
    participating in toxic relationships that are dragging you
    down, perhaps it's time to reassess and begin surrounding
    yourself with people who will help you move forward.

3. **Take time to plan.** Get your calendar out and plan time
    for activities that contribute to your health and wellness
    goals. Create some free time to work on this plan regularly,
    fine-tune your schedule, and make small shifts that will
    result in big changes over time.

4. **Get support.** Find your people. We all benefit from
    support and constructive input. I wouldn't have finished
    this book without support and accountability. Support
    allows us to stay motivated when all we want to do is sit
    on the couch and binge on Netflix, for example. A like-
    minded group also encourages us, cheers us on, and helps
    celebrate our successes. A *really* awesome group supports
    us through hard times, especially. That's when you know
    you've truly found your people.

5. **Be aware of how much you own (mentally and
    physically).** It takes time and money to manage clutter—
    whatever form it comes in. Maybe you need to literally
    lighten your load to be clearer on what you want and
    to more easily and effectively manage your day-to-day
    life. This may come in the form of creating a capsule
    wardrobe or clearing the kitchen counters to make it
    easy to prepare meals. Paper clutter can take up a lot
    of space too, both physically and mentally, so eliminate

the paper where you can by scanning, then discarding, old papers. Pretend you're moving! This is a great way to decide what stays and what goes. If you wouldn't pay to move it, then maybe it's time for a new home, whether that's the recycling bin, garbage, or the local Goodwill.

6. **Value your time.** Learn some tricks of the trade to end conversations and stay on track. My favorite is, "I would love to talk with you about this, but I've got an appointment. How about we catch up on Saturday morning?" Another is, "Let me think about it." This is a great way to say "no" without saying no in the moment, if that makes you uncomfortable. Then give yourself time, but be sure to follow up by saying, "I've given your offer some thought, but no thank you," or something else that feels right to you. (Don't feel the need to explain or lie to get out of something.) And show up—mostly for yourself. If you schedule time to exercise, then do it. If you schedule time for meal prep, make it happen.

7. **Implement effective systems**. Systems allow us to save time and energy. Truly! The major benefit of a system is that once in place, you get to fine-tune it. And over time, as you tweak the system, it runs more smoothly and efficiently. You can also teach a system to someone else. When you put systems in place at home and then teach them, it's really only necessary to oversee from there on out. Hopefully, at some point, you won't even have to supervise, just direct. If you have kids, you're also teaching them valuable life skills that will make them independent adults. You want them going off to college or out in the world knowing how to care for themselves, and that means doing their own laundry, shopping for groceries, and cleaning their own space. Take time to get these systems in place and teach others.

• Inner Critic •

Problems arise when we try to stay on course with change and our inner critic keeps rearing its ugly little head. The inner critic is the little voice that judges us, tells us we're not good enough, we can't do this, berates us when we make a mistake, creates confusion in our mind when we're on a good path and, ultimately, destroys our efforts. UNLESS we intervene and quiet the voice.

I first discovered my inner critic when I became a mom. I was already highly self-critical, but this was amplified when my first daughter was born. During my pregnancy, I read many books, so once my daughter was born and things didn't go exactly as planned, I became concerned that I wasn't doing motherhood correctly. I over-thought every decision and feared that I would make the wrong one. My inner critic was NOT helpful.

Since the average human has more than 60,000 thoughts each day, it's important to identify where at least some of those thoughts originated. As I mentioned earlier, a belief is a thought repeated again and again. These beliefs may come in the form of statements a well-meaning family member made when we were kids or from a teacher who, without knowing, instilled in us a thought pattern that we weren't good at math.

As an adult, our first boss could've been negative and challenging in a bad way. Or we could have been part of an organization or community that we later discovered just didn't fit our way of thinking.

Repeated thoughts that make us feel bad and sometimes feel physically heavy. Our *inner critic* can grow over many years and become the primary ruler of our mind. An easy way to spot the difference between our inner critic and true authentic self is this: The inner critic makes us feel bad, lethargic, and is heavy in our body. When we are our true, authentic self, we tend to be light, breathe easier and feel confident in our thinking.

Keep in mind that when we attempt to make change in our thinking, there will be setbacks. That's perfectly normal. Things may even become a little messy. The inner critic can rear its ugly head and overload us with every negative thought we've ever had about ourselves. But staying conscious and aware while dismissing the negativity is key in making progress.

• The Broccoli Incident •

My dad died suddenly when I was five years old. After that, I grew up in a single-parent home. I'm the oldest of three, with a twenty-three month difference between my sister and me and only eleven months in between my sister and younger brother. As a teenager, it was largely the responsibility of my sister and me to start dinner before our mom came home from work, while my brother somehow got away with lying on the couch and watching TV. *Hmmmmm.*

One night, as we prepared dinner, my sister asked me to steam the broccoli. Up to this point, there had never been any real instruction on how to steam broccoli; my sister just seemed to know what to do or was a very good improviser. Being the oldest, I didn't want to look like I didn't know what I was doing, so I grabbed a pot, dropped the broccoli in, added a little water, put it on the stove, covered it with a lid, turned the gas to medium, and went about my business (probably doing homework).

Just as my mom walked in the door from work, my sister yelled, "Oh my God, you've burned the broccoli!" She grabbed the pot and tossed it in the sink. My mother chimed in too, "You burned the broccoli."

Well, in that moment, I was not only banished from the kitchen, but from that day on, anytime I offered to help, the "you burned the broccoli" mantra was repeated and I was dismissed.

Looking back, it was pretty funny, given the expectation that a person's cooking abilities were defined at a time when they actually had no skills. This incident did get me off the hook for serious kitchen duties, but it stifled my confidence for many years.

The broccoli incident, however, created anxiety surrounding cooking for most of my adult life. I wasn't even aware that it was that specific incident that haunted me. However, every time I'd get in the kitchen, I would unconsciously doubt my abilities and was never happy or satisfied with how and what I cooked for my family.

I share this for two reasons. First, we need to be careful how we speak to others because we don't truly understand or know the long-lasting impact our words can have on people. Second, we need to identify our own beliefs about ourselves that keep us stuck so we can change those beliefs and move forward to create success.

Interestingly, I've raised two daughters who, in spite of my negative childhood experience, are amazing foodies who can shop, prepare, and cook awesome meals for themselves and others. So patterns can be broken!

• Shifting Negative Beliefs •

Now let's move on to shifting the negative beliefs that interfere with our goal of a healthy lifestyle.

The degree of negative thoughts vary for everyone, and some beliefs are more obvious than others. However, whether conscious or not, we can all fine-tune our thinking. I encourage you to work through the exercises at the end of this chapter to support you in creating a solid foundation for permanent change.

Although I've described a belief as a thought we think over and over again, let's define it more accurately here: "an acceptance that a statement is true or that something exists; trust, faith, or confidence in someone or something."

Women, in particular, have thoughts about themselves and their bodies that include:

"I can't lose weight no matter how much I try."

"I've always been heavy. My mother was heavy."

"I just love sweets."

"I *only* drink DIET soda."

These untruths are things we've come to believe and accept, but when we unconsciously internalize them, they hold us back.

If nothing else, an attempt to shift or change our beliefs leads to a greater understanding of ourselves. I will warn you, however, that as you change your beliefs about yourself and the world around you, it's possible that relationships will shift, friendships will change, and some people may drop out of your life. Why? Well, as we gain more confidence in ourselves, feel more comfortable expressing who we are, and demonstrate greater self-love, other people get uncomfortable because it naturally requires them to look at themselves. And if they're not up for the task, they may retaliate with sarcasm or criticism or they may stop returning phone calls or texts.

Although this can be confusing, awkward, and uncomfortable, it's a sign that you are becoming stronger and getting to know yourself more deeply. So hang in there and keep moving forward to create the healthiest you. Those who also want to grow will come along for the ride.

• Self-Compassion: The Key to Long-Lasting, Permanent Change •

As you move through the process of identifying your beliefs and work through shifting them, it's important to demonstrate self-compassion. The essence of self-compassion is to love yourself.

Here we go again with a definition. Self-compassion is "compassion towards one's self in instances of perceived inadequacy, failure, or general suffering."

Who hasn't experienced failure or suffering? I know I have, and in many of those moments, I was unkind and even mean to myself, not demonstrating any level of self-compassion. Instead, I berated myself and told myself in so many words that I wasn't good enough.

When I first became aware of the idea of self-compassion, I

began to think of my children and a specific incident that involved my youngest daughter.

My daughters and I were on a road trip one summer, driving home after visiting family in another state. We were 500 miles into the 800-mile trip. I was tired and couldn't wait to get home. We stopped at a rest area to use the facilities and grab drinks. As we got back on the road, my youngest daughter, who was about six at the time and buckled into her car seat, spilled her entire container of milk. The whole thing! All over her and the backseat. I pulled the car over, got out of the car to clean her up, but I was so frustrated that I proceeded to yell at her. She stared at me, wide-eyed. I realized in that moment that I was frightening her. I stopped, but I felt horrible, guilty, and ashamed and wondered if she would ever forgive me.

I was NOT demonstrating compassion. She was six, and she spilled milk.

I'm not perfect and I have been frustrated with my children more than a time or two, but I used that incident as a reminder to shift my reactions and how I spoke with them. Then, unknowingly at first, I used this same incident as a reminder to shift how I would speak to myself moving forward. If I wouldn't speak to people I love in a mean and berating manner, why would I do that to myself? I don't deserve that and neither do you.

When we demonstrate self-compassion, we learn to become our own best friend. Sounds a little corny, perhaps. However, we're the only constant in our lives so we need to learn to rely on being kind to ourselves. We must parent ourselves. It's an inside job!

I've found that demonstrating self-love, kindness, patience, and forgiveness toward myself changes everything. The inner critic quiets and I can breathe easier and forgive myself more quickly.

Sometimes the process doesn't happen as quickly as I'd like. There are times when I have made an error in judgment or hurt someone's feelings but didn't realize it until later. And perhaps that person wasn't ready to talk about it or accept an apology, so I've had to sit through the uncomfortable feelings and wait it out. It's humbling to sit with pain and still move forward with what needs to get done when there's an unresolved matter looming.

If we attempt to "fix" things too quickly, we can miss the point and the opportunity to heal on a level that's much deeper and more permanent. With awareness and acceptance of our behavior, sitting with the pain can transform us and help lead us to greater emotional growth. And with emotional growth comes less stress and more confidence.

Society today is set up for people to find validation and love outside themselves. Apparently, it's in the clothing we buy or the awesome selfies we take. If we watch mainstream TV or spend time on sites that contain consumer advertising (which is everywhere now), we are constantly told that for people to love us, we need a particular type of hairstyle or makeup. We need to drive a certain car, carry a particular bag, and have a particular type of partner who also does all of those things. It's exhausting and we have it all wrong.

Those are life's distractions from what's really important, what really matters, and the journey of finding out who we truly are.

When we demonstrate kindness to ourselves in the way we would to loved ones, we create a softness within ourselves that echoes out to people and the world around us.

When we understand that self-compassion and self-love are what we truly need, and we have the ability to give that to ourselves, we can begin to share that with others. This is the beginning of what changes the world around us.

Over the years, I've found that in order to create and sustain any permanent change in my life, it's critical to practice self-compassion. When we're gentle with ourselves, we're more easily able to accept our flaws, our procrastination, the ways we've sabotaged ourselves in the past, and begin to forgive ourselves and move forward like we've never done before.

• Exercise 1: Shifting Beliefs that No Longer Serve Us •

For many, the negative self-talk may be a bit insidious, meaning that you are completely unaware of what you say to yourself because ignoring or tuning it out has become a habit and a pattern deeply ingrained. For example, you may have unconscious mantras that you repeat to yourself specifically surrounding how you think about your body.

Be brave, know you're not alone, and take some time to sit quietly before proceeding with this exercise. Recall a time when you were upset with yourself or something someone else did that put you into a funk or a tailspin. Recall what you were thinking and saying in your mind. Were you replaying over and over what you *should* have said? Instead of focusing on the issues, were you more hung up on berating yourself?

Asking yourself these questions may have brought up some heavy emotions. That means you're on the right track to more deeply discovering your inner critic. Awareness is the first key, so good job!

WHAT ARE YOUR CURRENT BELIEFS?

Now let's move on to shifting some negative beliefs. As mentioned earlier in the chapter, our beliefs typically stem from something we learned or heard and then internalized. Perhaps when we were growing up, our parents meant well, but instilled fear in us by saying something like, "Well, you can try gymnastics, but it's going to be really hard." Then you tried and didn't succeed in the way you thought you would and decided not to continue, so it became your belief that not only was gymnastics hard, but other things probably were too so you stopped trying.

Another example is the belief that you can't lose weight. That may have come from a well-meaning mom who repeated that mantra because that's what her mom said. Or from that saying from many moons ago, "A second on the lips and a lifetime on the hips." Again, perhaps a well-meaning saying, but one that had you considering every piece of food you put in your mouth from then on.

So, take a deep breath and begin to think about some of the beliefs you have about yourself. We're talking primarily negative beliefs here because they're the ones you want to shift. However, do make a note of some of the positive beliefs you have, too. This can help when this feels tough.

Making this list will come easy for some just by thinking of people closest to you. Before I resolved some negative beliefs I had, I could pretty quickly identify them just by thinking of a particular person in my life because the thought of them would immediately have me repeating over and over in my head what that person thought of me. Fortunately, there are not too many people like that in my life (especially now) but there was a time when the list was longer.

Example: "I CAN'T lose weight no matter how hard I try."

List your negative beliefs here (and grab a journal or a piece of paper if you have more than five that you want to explore):

1.
2.
3.
4.
5.

LET'S CREATE NEW BELIEFS!

Now let's work through creating what will be positive replacement beliefs that can be used as affirmations or mantras as you begin to adopt them. Take each one from above and reframe the belief into a positive phrase or statement. This may require you to write something that doesn't resonate with you currently, especially if it's a deep-seated belief, but do it anyway.

EXAMPLE of revised belief: "I lose weight easily and maintain my ideal weight with little effort."

1.

2.

3.

4.

5.

Begin to say these new beliefs out loud at least a couple of times each day. Write them on sticky notes and place them on the bathroom mirror or write them on index cards and put them on the fridge. When you catch yourself talking negatively to yourself or repeating a negative belief, STOP and repeat the positive replacement.

Great work! You dug deep. This is no easy task, so pat yourself on the back and continue to practice self-care.

• Exercise 2: Exploring & Embracing Self-Compassion •

EXPLORING SELF-COMPASSION

Now it's time to recall a scenario when you did NOT demonstrate self-compassion in a particular situation. For example, you had a disagreement with a friend and in your mind, over and over, you called yourself names or spoke negatively to yourself because you. felt you could have handled the situation better. Or you were feeling stretched for time and weren't very nice to the grocery store clerk who didn't have the item you needed for a recipe. The purpose of this is to consciously identify a specific example in order to change it and other instances where you were unkind to yourself.

Journal below the circumstances of the situation, how you felt, your thoughts, and any statements you made to yourself about what transpired.

-    Circumstances (write a brief description of the situation):

_____

_____

_____

_____

_____

-    How you felt (for example, fearful, full of self-doubt,
     upset, confused):

_____

_____

_____

_____

_____

-    Thoughts surrounding the situation:

_____

_____

_____

_____

-    How you spoke to yourself about what transpired:

_____

_____

_____

_____

- What could you have done differently in the situation? How could you have demonstrated self-compassion? Think in terms of what you said to yourself during and after the situation, how you treated yourself emotionally, how you treated your physical body, and how you treated others as a result of the situation. What you would tell someone you love and care for—your best friend or child—and how would you speak to them?

_____

_____

_____

_____

_____

_____

_____

_____

_____

_____

Note: use the above prompts to explore any additional situations you repeatedly replay in your mind, whether it was a disagreement with a family or friend, a situation where you were dissatisfied with how someone treated you or maybe something that you continually repeat in your mind over and over again.

PRACTICING SELF-COMPASSION

Now let's look at how you can be gentler and kinder to yourself.

What negative language can you eliminate from your vocabulary that is currently not supporting your efforts to express self-compassion? For example, ask yourself, _Am I using negative phrases or words such as "this always happens to me" or "I can't" or "I'll never" statements._

Using words like *always* or *never* can block the flow of any positivity surrounding your efforts. Therefore, it's important to eliminate these negative words. See the Resources section for a book recommendation ("A Complaint Free World" by Will Bowen) that can offer help if this is an on-going and truly challenging issue.

List five negative words or phrases you say to yourself regularly:

1.
2.
3.
4.
5.

Now list five positive words or phrases that you could replace the above with:

1.
2.
3.
4.
5.

How can you demonstrate self-compassion on a daily basis? For example: repeating positive mantras and affirmations to yourself, speaking up for yourself, drinking less or no caffeine, eliminating sugar, exercising and movement, quiet time, practicing positive self-talk.

List at least five ways you can begin to demonstrate self-compassion:

1.
2.
3.
4.
5.

How do you think your daily life will change as a result of
practicing self-compassion?

_____

_____

_____

_____

_____

_____

_____

_____

_____

_____

_____

• Exercise 3: Mindful Eating •

Life is busy, and at meal time, many people and families wind up
scrolling through their phones or eating meals while watching TV.
Without even realizing it, they gobble down a meal, not having
thoroughly tasted or enjoyed it.

Mindful eating involves focusing on the food and enjoying
what you're eating; noticing the tastes, textures, and enjoyment
surrounding the food. There's even research that shows you eat less
and more slowly when you eat mindfully because you're tasting and
focusing on the food.

Follow this exercise to eat more mindfully:

1. **Focus on the preparation.** Prepare your meal without
   the usual distractions. Turn off the TV, turn off the ringer
   on your phone. Enjoy the task of preparing and cooking.

2. **Set the table.** Create a space where you can sit and enjoy your food without distractions or disruptions.

3. **Bless your food.** Whether you're religious, spiritual, agnostic, or atheist, be thankful for your food and be mindful to acknowledge that before you eat.

4. **Taste your food.** Studies show that it's actually the first bite that tastes the best, not the last. Savor the flavors and allow yourself to truly enjoy what you're eating.

5. **Chew slowly.** When you chew slowly, this will allow for easier and better digestion.

Other ways to create a mindful eating experience include scheduling dinner with family or friends a specific number of times each week in which you prepare a meal together, sit and eat leisurely, and clean up together. Note: if you're a family with sporting activities that take place during "dinner time," be sure to prep in advance so you're not hitting the drive-through.

What are some ways that you can practice mindful eating?

_____

_____

_____

_____

_____

_____

• Mindless vs. Mindful •

Mindless: Not recognizing that our unmonitored thoughts dictate the outcome of our daily efforts.

Mindful: Creating space to recognize our thoughts and beliefs, then changing what we know isn't getting us the results we want.

We can't forget that in order to be truly healthy, we must move our bodies. Our body is our vehicle that transports us on a daily basis. To show its appreciation, we must move it, move it. Let's move onto Chapter 3 where we'll dive into exercise and movement.

CHAPTER 3

Easy Exercise & Movement

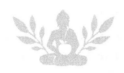

Some movement is better than none, so get up and dance!

• Early Movement •

One of my earliest memories of physical exercise takes place in a dance and tumbling class at a studio above a deli in the center of the small town where I grew up. I remember wearing a black, short-sleeved leotard, white tights and black ballet flats with my hair in a bun on the top of my head.

This introduction to movement helped me remain active as I was growing up. My neighborhood friends and I spent hours outdoors, running around doing cartwheels and handsprings. We didn't have the distractions of technology and Netflix, and in the 1970s, most parents told kids to go outside and play and we did—for hours. Oftentimes, not returning home until the streetlights came on. Different times.

In my early years, I was also a member of a 4-H baton twirling squad, practicing once a week and participating in town parades. Again, this kept me outdoors and active; you couldn't toss a baton too high indoors without getting in trouble.

In middle school, I played recreational softball. I was on a team—

the Red Sox—with friends from another neighborhood, while my sister and best friend played on the Yankees, which included many kids from our neighborhood. I'm not exactly how this happened, but it was kind of disappointing because my sister and best friend's team won a lot and the coach had a cool convertible she'd drive her winning team around in. The coach would honk the horn while the winning players waived their yellow caps. But being on a team was fun, and I learned a lot about teamwork and my physical capabilities. I played various positions, from shortstop to third base and occasionally pitcher.

Around the same time, I briefly ran track too, but again didn't embrace what running could do for my body. I quickly went from running the mile to twenty-five-meter dash, then lost interest.

In high school, I attempted to revive my short-lived track experience and even tried out for softball, but both of these went by the wayside, and I no longer experienced movement on a regular basis. It was around this time that my anxiety began to show up in ways I hadn't experienced previously. I also hadn't discovered yet that health really begins from the inside out. In other words, you can look good on the outside but still not feel good on the inside.

And easily maintaining a "healthy" weight did not serve me well. I ignored what I was putting in my body and most of the time felt foggy and sluggish due to the combination of poor nutrients and no regular exercise.

This would be the case for many years to come.

I became incredibly self-conscious when it came to the act of exercising, and my anxiety continued to worsen. When someone invited me to exercise—running, going to the gym, or participating in a class—I felt self-conscious and awkward. Occasionally, I'd push myself, but then I would retreat because I felt overwhelmed and uncomfortable. I didn't know how to work through this awkward stage and never pushed through to the other side where I could gain a regular routine to help me naturally reduce stress and release the endorphins—the happy hormones.

I would occasionally play tennis, go biking or rollerblading, and use at-home workout videos. But there was no consistent effort, even though deep down I knew exercise and movement was the answer to feeling better. It just seemed easier to sort of hide from it.

By my mid-twenties, I had somewhat convinced myself that medication would help me get to a place in my mind so that I could exercise consistently. An antidepressant lifted my mood somewhat, but it didn't get me moving. I did, however, feel a little less anxious.

Although I engaged in spurts of indoor exercising (including step aerobics, which annoyed my downstairs neighbor to the point he offered to buy me a pair of fleece-lined slippers), I still didn't incorporate regular and consistent movement into my life.

Daily movement is beneficial, but for many—myself included—this doesn't happen because we don't build it into our schedules or we just don't feel like it. Some of us just think it's not possible for us. We're anxious or self-conscious about stepping into a studio or gym, or we just don't know where to start. I used both excuses.

When it comes to exercise, there's good news and bad news. The bad news is most of us won't ever say, "I can't wait to go to the gym." The good news is that when we put in the work and gain momentum and motivation, going to the gym becomes easier and more desirable.

Exercise is an import part of losing weight. But it also contributes to a healthier mind and body. And remember: past behavior doesn't have to predict future behavior.

• Inconsistency Continues •

I married in my late twenties, and together, we didn't do a very good job of creating a regular exercise routine. Movement improved once I had children because the kids were walking and wanted to be outside. But this movement was more bending and chasing versus focused workouts.

What was consistent, however, were the negative statements and questions I had repeated to myself for years, which included:

You know movement is the answer.
Why don't you make a commitment and follow through
every day?
Why can't you do this?
You should be able to do this!
You probably can't do this, anyway.

And my favorite way of showing self-love was to remind myself constantly that if I had just put in the effort when I was younger I wouldn't be in this predicament now. Self-flagellation and berating myself constantly, without consciously realizing it.

• Finally, a Shift •

Several years later (did I mention this was a long journey?) I'd had enough of feeling unappreciative of myself. I was in my early forties, happily divorced, but still completely overwhelmed with the stress of daily life that included raising children as a single mom. I read self-help books and attended workshops that helped with my mindset a lot, but I still wasn't moving my body regularly. I blamed it on the weather, I blamed it on not having enough time, and I finally admitted to myself that I just wasn't doing it.

However, I knew in my gut that movement was the answer to reducing and possibly eliminating anxiety all together. That nagging little voice at the back of my head—that voice of reason—wouldn't stop.

Finally, I decided to go to the gym! It was really as simple as that and this was a major turning point. At the time, one of the local gyms only cost ten dollars a month. That's $2.50 a week. Less than I spent on one grande caramel macchiato at Starbucks, which I also cut out. I got on the treadmill. I ran until I felt like I was going to throw up, then slowed to a walk. Then I increased my speed, ran for a few minutes, then walked again. This went on for thirty minutes, which is what I committed to that day. I did it! I finished thirty minutes of self-inflicted torture, but I did it.

I went back again two days later and did the same thing, only each time I returned for another session, I ran for longer periods, improving my overall mile per hour pace. After the first week of going to the gym four times, I felt really optimistic (or I was just ignorant) and signed up for the annual 10K race in my town, which has grown to more than 40,000 runners. I'm goal-oriented, so this helped me focus and persevere. I now had less than three months to "learn" how to run about six miles at one time.

Dealing with anxiety hasn't been an easy process, by any means. Sometimes it felt like a moment-to-moment struggle. Sometimes all I could do was to tell my anxiety to shut up. Eventually I learned that what I needed to do was make friends with my anxiety because the likelihood of it going away entirely was slim, no matter how much I moved my body. But I managed to get to a place where I've learned to live with it.

Some days I feel okay and my anxiety is under control, but other days, especially when I've had too much coffee or have too many things on the calendar, I get irritated and annoyed. For a moment, anxiety is in charge. May sound a little unusual to those who haven't experienced anxiety, but for those who have, it probably makes sense. And for those who don't experience it, count your blessings.

• Mind over Matter •

So back to running. I always told myself I can't run, along with many other "can't" statements. The truth was I could run. I just needed to work at it.

Other runners will likely understand too that the experience of running is oftentimes a mind game. Sometimes, setting small goals like making it to the next street corner or to keep going for another two minutes is all you need to reach your next level. Then you run two more minutes and realize that you can keep going. When you do this repeatedly, you build strength and confidence. It's very gratifying.

After only a month of running, I was feeling better overall and stronger in both mind and body.

Less than three months after I started running, I finished the 10K I signed up for in 1:06:58, a respectable time for a first-timer.

The night before the race, I felt like it was the night before the first day of school. I had my new clothes laid out and my alarm set to get up at zero-dark-thirty (it was early!). I was exhilarated and excited. I was also anxious, but with a few months of running behind me, I also felt confident and knew I would finish.

Several weeks after finishing the 10K, the Universe brought me a running partner. This was unexpected and helped me take running to another level.

• The Impact of Accountability •

My running partner showed up at the bus stop after school one day when we were both picking up our daughters. Susie was wearing running clothes, and after figuring out that we both ran, we scheduled a time to run later that week. Until then, I had been running at the gym on a treadmill. With the exception of the 10K, I was a treadmill runner. Susie, on the other hand, was a street and trail runner who, I later came to find out, had been running for twenty-five years, completing eight marathons and a few triathlons during that time. Talk about being intimidated and anxious—it was good I didn't know or was too ignorant to realize she was a seasoned athlete.

Susie was supportive, patient, and encouraging. After running together two to three times a week for about seven months, she called one day to see if I'd be interested in running a half marathon in Jacksonville, Florida. What? A half marathon? Up to that point, the farthest I had run was about six miles at one time, and the half marathon was only six weeks away. After slightly wrapping my brain around what would be involved, I said yes. Again, some ignorance here.

For the next six weeks, we upped our mileage, running at least five times a week for four to five miles each run; on the weekends, we did longer runs. The Saturday before the half marathon, I ran ten miles in preparation, which was the longest run I had ever accomplished in one session. On February 17, 2013, I finished the half marathon in 2:09:07.

Another game changer for my health and an example of how I began to increase self-esteem and confidence.

• Transitions •

In 2015, I transitioned to yoga, which had been on my list for a long time, but similar to going to the gym, I was intimidated to enter a yoga studio. But knew I could manage this transition because I had done it with running.

I found an amazing yoga community and adopted a regular form of meditation that helped me further my personal growth. Meditation is proven to reduce stress and anxiety and increase brain function, and the breathing aspect helps reduce high blood pressure and improve circulation due to deep, steady, controlled breathing. I received all those benefits!

When working out became part of my lifestyle, I began eating healthier and eliminating toxic relationships in my life. To my surprise, my outlook on life changed dramatically. Suddenly I had more purpose. I met healthier people in social groups, and they also had health goals. Most importantly, I felt more at home in my head and body than I ever had.

Today, a laundry hamper full of dirty workout clothes represents a good week.

• The Body Needs Love •

Exercise and movement are huge acts of self-compassion. In the previous chapter, we talked about ways to reduce the busy-ness. But whether we slow down or not, movement in our everyday lives is crucial to living a healthier lifestyle.

I love what Gene Tunney, a World Heavyweight Champion in the 1920s, said about exercise: "Exercise should be regarded as a tribute to the heart." Both literally and figuratively. The heart is the instrument that keeps our body functioning—it needs solid, healthy breathing to keep blood circulating. And it's the blood that flows through it that helps maintain a healthy heart.

We also need to love our heart because it's where we feel emotion.

I don't know about you, but there were times when my heart was broken. When I feel down or disappointed, nothing helps more than deep, steady breathing and a long walk to get the body moving and keep the heart pumping optimally.

Our bodies carry emotions. Our posture can also have an impact on how we feel. And, unfortunately, with today's over use of smartphones, we are often in a position of having our head down, which likely affects our mood. When people are depressed, they often have their head in a downward position. However, if you notice people who are typically positive and optimistic, their posture is usually upright and their body movements, especially their head, reflect a "let's get moving" attitude.

• Instantly Change How You Feel •

If you're lacking energy and feeling a little blah but don't have time for a quick walk, a full workout or even a call with a good friend who knows how to snap you out of it, there are ways to shift your emotions. Simply putting a smile on your face can help, but that may be a stretch, depending upon the emotion you're experiencing at the time. Here's a little mood boosting that you could even do in the bathroom stall at work because it doesn't require a whole lot of room:

1. Stand up with legs hip-distance apart and arms straight up in a "V" position.

2. Keep your posture straight and head tilted up slightly.
3. Breathe deeply and slowly through your nose, smile (not necessary) and hold this for two minutes.

You'll begin to feel some energy swirl throughout your body. If possible, take a quick lap around the house or office to continue blood flow. Do this on a regular basis and you'll crave this method to help you feel better instantly after too much screen time, too much work at a desk or if you receive an unpleasant text or get stuck in a traffic jam.

The small shifts really do get big results, so think about how you can incorporate movement during your everyday activities. For example, there's no reason you can't move about while you're brushing your teeth. Ideally, we want to brush our teeth for two minutes anyway to promote healthy oral hygiene, so instead of being annoyed that you have to brush for two minutes, work in some movement too. Dance it out and get in some squats!

When you're making healthy meals, use that time to take a twirl, do some leg lifts, and take a walk around the kitchen in between tasks.

• Determining What Works For You •

Identifying what makes you move is important. Let's face it, the studio and the gym are not for everyone. If you're an introvert like me, being around a lot of other people who are lifting weights, dancing, etc. can deplete your energy. We introverts know that we do best re-energizing when we are typically at home or in a quiet place. So you may do better in a private or semi-private class, going to the gym during off hours, running outdoors alone or with a small group, or even a yoga class where you stay on a mat and can close your eyes.

Studios and gyms are a great place for extroverts, who tend to re-energize by being around other people. So if you get energized that way, consider classes like Zumba, spinning, or working out in a crowded gym. You'll likely do best with an activity that is higher energy with opportunities to engage other people.

The energy of the group can make a difference and help you to push yourself a little more than you might if left on your own. This goes for both introverts and extroverts. Either way, incorporating movement can be as simple as pulling out your laptop, iPad, or smartphone and opening a YouTube video. There's truly no reason not to get started. Have fun doing the research, but limit yourself to how long you have to find an activity so you DO get moving.

If you do best with support and accountability, factor that into your decision when it comes to choosing the activity, the place, and the time.

Use the exercise called "What Makes You Move" at the end of this chapter to determine what works best for you. This will take you through a series of questions to help you identify what works for you when it comes to movement.

• How to Get Moving •

- Find your why. Having a why works sort of like a guidance system. It's what we're aiming for. In the midst of attempting to reach any type of goal without a target or a why, we can get off course and wind up somewhere else, or just lose focus all together. Therefore, defining your why early will help get you exactly where you want to be. So when it comes to your health, explore your why for wanting to get healthier. Is it to lower cholesterol, lose weight, or improve relationships? There's no right or wrong answer—your why is your why—just define it.

- Schedule it. Use the exercise in this chapter to define when you will exercise, then stick to it. Just like a doctor, nail, or hair appointment, put exercise and movement on your calendar.

- Create accountability. Maybe it's a well-meaning friend (not the one who will invite you out for a beer and say, "Ah, don't worry about it, you can start next week") or a personal trainer or simply showing up for a class. Find a friend, coach, or trainer who will support you in reaching your health goals.

- Incorporate non-food-related rewards. This may be treating yourself to a massage after you've reached a certain goal or a new fitness outfit in a smaller size. Something that doesn't cost much and contributes to future success.

- Under promise, over deliver. This is one of the most valuable lessons I have learned, and it applies to many areas of life. I've used it in business and in my personal life, and I recommend to clients that they adopt this philosophy when it comes to their own personal wellness journey. Set a smaller goal and surpass it! When you do this, psychologically you can experience many positive effects.

- Don't wait for the perfect time because there is no such thing. Start today!

- Do something—anything is movement. Ten squats standing in your kitchen is better than nothing.

• Create a New Routine •

Often we are in a cycle that's not serving us and we simply need to break it.

Have you ever had to take a detour from your typical driving route to work or the grocery store due to a traffic jam or road construction? All of a sudden you're not on auto-pilot and you needing to pay attention to the direction you're headed. Same goes for other routines. We drive to and from work, sometimes not even remembering how we got there, but we did because we took the same route we've taken for the last two years.

Changing up your routine is one of the best ways to incorporate a change in habit. For example, instead of heading directly home after work—we all know that once we arrive home, getting back out the door to the gym or studio is challenging—go directly from work.

• Visible Reminders •

Unless something is directly in front of us, we may not take notice. I love an uncluttered home, but sometimes to remember something, it needs to be literally in front of me or under my feet. I'll place my re-packed gym bag on the floor at the front door so I don't forget it or place my sneakers in the hallway so I have to trip over them.

Visible reminders are a great way to stay motivated. Here are some suggestions:

- Put an inspiring quote on your fridge.
- Put a screensaver on your smartphone.
- Place an unrolled yoga mat in your living area.
- Put your running shoes by the front door.
- Place a packed gym bag on the front seat of your car.

Check your surroundings periodically to make sure your visible reminders haven't become permanent fixtures (for example, weights that are now used as a doorstop). If that has happened, reassess whether it's the right activity or consider whether your home could use a little decluttering. We'll talk about that more later.

These visible reminders may take time to equate to action, but they will serve a purpose as you work toward incorporating more movement into your daily life.

• Movement at Work •

There's no easy way to say this, so I'll just put it out there: desk jobs are the worst for our overall health! It's pretty common knowledge that sitting is the new smoking. I had a desk job for years and wondered why I felt tired and achy at the end of the day.

To create more movement at work:

- **Incorporate a standup desk.** This is a great way to strengthen your legs, your posture and gain more movement. You can do lunges, leg lifts and squeeze your buttocks, rotate your ankles, do overhead arm stretches.

- **Take a break.** Get up at least once an hour and take a lap around the office, refill your water bottle, allow your eyes to focus on something in the distance, and say a cheerful *hello* to someone else in the office. If you work from home, go outside and say hello to a neighbor.

- **Eat lunch.** Move away from your desk and practice mindful eating, go for a walk outside, get some fresh air.

- **Relocate.** If your workplace has a kitchen area or high-top table, take your laptop and stand up for a while. Working from home? Take your laptop outdoors or to another room.

Many companies are encouraging employees to get more movement during their day by taking a walk or by providing standing desks. If your company doesn't already offer a wellness program, talk with human resources to see how you could help move them in that direction.

• Get Outdoors •

Weather permitting, this is probably the easiest option when it comes to movement. Grab your sneakers and take a stroll. Breathe the fresh air, enjoy the sunshine. Or if it's cold, bundle up. The cold can wake you up and make you feel more energized.

Other simple and accessible outdoor activities include running and biking. And there are many fitness groups and trainers who offer Pilates in the park, yoga at the beach, or Zumba on the playground. With a little Googling or Facebooking, you'll find all sorts of options in your area. Also, try Meetup.com. This is a great site to find people who have similar interests.

• Support and Accountability •

Critical to any success is support and accountability. Think of a time when you were required to check in on a particular activity or project. We tend to achieve more when we have a cheering section. I could not have completed this book without the support and accountability of a writing coach. Meeting deadlines and completing the work would have taken longer if I didn't have to check in with someone who had my back.

In addition, the feedback and kudos are helpful when we're trying to achieve something we've never done before or have been challenged by in the past.

When choosing an accountability partner, choose someone who will help you stay on track and refocus when you get off track, because that happens—it's part of the process. You also want someone who can provide honest feedback in a way that resonates with you to keep you moving forward.

We all need support in every area of our lives, and when it comes to being healthier, I can't stress this enough. So start thinking about who can support you and ask for their help today.

Here are the exercises for this chapter. I encourage you to complete each one, which will help identify the best type of exercise for you, develop a routine, and create a schedule that works for you.

• Exercise 1: What Makes You Move •

In this exercise, you'll think about what's happening now and where you'd like to be. This is to create a solid goal and track progress as you head toward it.

Let's begin with the NOW.

What type of movement/exercise activities are you currently doing?

_____

_____

How many days a week do you currently exercise?

_____

_____

Now let's figure out what will get you moving. Think about what really gets you going! (Note: if you're already clear on that, move on to how you can create more movement and/or what are you willing to commit to.)

For some people, Zumba is ideal because of the music combined with the movement, as well as the energy of other people in the room.

For others, going to a gym, plugging in headphones, and getting on the treadmill for thirty minutes is their thing.

And for others, yoga might be their form of movement—and within yoga, there are different options, from restorative to yin to hot yoga.

In this chapter, we talked about how introverts and extroverts might choose their type of exercising and movement activities. If you prefer to exercise in a group or in the privacy of your own home, that's fine. The key is to move your body, so choose what resonates with you.

Let's identify specifics. Just list what first comes to mind. If you're having trouble coming up with examples, I've provided some for inspiration.

What makes you move? (Is it music, other people's energy, time
of day?)

_____

_____

_____

_____

What can you do to create more movement? (For example, walk
your dog, take the stairs, do squats while preparing dinner.)

_____

_____

_____

_____

What are you willing to commit to? (For example, thirty minutes
a day, three times a week). You decide but be realistic based on
the other commitments you have in your life. Remember, under
promise, over deliver!

_____

_____

_____

_____

• Exercise 2: Developing Your Exercise Routine •

Now it's time to develop a routine of movement that works for you
personally, including time of day, type of movement, frequency, and
enjoyment level.

Ideally, you want to move every day, whether it's simply taking the stairs versus the elevator, a full workout or something in between. Remember, oftentimes you can work in movement without having to formally schedule it, which include things like taking the stairs, returning the shopping cart back inside the store (you'll get rewarded with extra karma points too), parking farther away than necessary from where you are headed.

Opportunities to move exist everywhere.

Sometimes it takes some conscious thought about how we execute our daily schedule. One way to wake up to a new way of doing something is driving a different route to work or the supermarket the next time you go out. You can do this without a GPS for added awareness. You'll notice different sights, sounds, and maybe even smells. Too often, we become unconscious and lost in unproductive thought, so it's time to change that.

Think about your daily schedule, then write down how you could incorporate more movement into your life:

SUPPORT SYSTEM

Creating a support system (a.k.a. accountability) is important when we're trying to achieve goals, whether a cheerleader-like family member or friend, someone who exercises with you, or a personal trainer or coach.

You also want to avoid the naysayers who don't hold us accountable when we ask them to or when you give excuses, they also make excuses for you. These people may be well-meaning, but as soon as you express that you'd rather stay home and eat pizza, they pick up the phone and order one for you.

Turn to people you can rely on for firm but consistent support.

Who is supportive of your desire to incorporate more movement in your life?

_____

_____

_____

_____

_____

_____

Identifying the qualities of a good support person or system can help you expand that support by looking for the same qualities in other people. This may come in the form of a person at work you hadn't considered before or maybe it's a neighbor. Important thing is to think about the qualities that are attractive to you when it comes to making progress in the area of movement and exercise.

What are the qualities about this person or group that inspires you?

_____

_____

_____

_____

_____

BODY INFORMATION

If weight loss isn't a concern for you, or you don't own a scale, not a big deal. How we feel is more important than the number, and by making healthier food choices, we naturally shed excess weight through a reduction in bloating and inflammation.

But if the number is important for tracking progress, enter it below.

Current weight?

_____

Are you happy with that weight? Why or why not?
(If not, include a goal weight in your goal.)

_____

_____

_____

_____

What types of physical limitations, if any, are you currently experiencing?

_____

_____

_____

_____

If you are experiencing physical limitations, always check with your doctor if you've been advised to either refrain from or limit physical activity.

Now let's move to Exercise 3 to create the schedule.

• Exercise 3: Creating an Exercise Schedule •

Exercise is done for many reasons, but the main one is to improve how we feel. When we exert ourselves physically, the body's opiate receptors activate, naturally making us feel better. The body also produces dopamine and endorphins, and these two combine to reduce stress and increase our level of contentment.

• Creating Change •

In order to make change, it's necessary to set realistic goals and break them down into manageable steps, keeping in mind that it's the small shifts that result in big changes over time. I encourage you to do something small and incorporate it in your regular schedule to make it a habit. Then add something else you'd like to change.

> *"A goal without a plan is just a wish."*
> —ANTOINE DE SAINT-EXUPÉRY

Now it's time to commit to a movement or exercise routine, because without commitment, it likely won't happen.

Let's start here:

1. What did you identify as an activity/exercise that would get you moving (we did this in Exercise 1: What Makes You Move?):

2. How much time are you willing to commit each week (for example, three thirty-minute sessions or two forty-five-minute sessions)? This is totally up to you and your schedule—remember under promise, over deliver.

---

3. Does this exercise involve signing up for a class or gym? Yes/No

   If No, move onto #4

   If Yes, do you have a history of signing up but not showing up? Yes/No

   If Yes, then do you want to reconsider something that would NOT incur the expense? Yes/No

   If Yes, the go back to #1. If No, then proceed to #4.

4. Choose your support person. Contact them, tell them your intentions, asking for accountability.

---

5. Take out your calendar and schedule time to exercise or move.

This is very important. Unless we schedule and prepare, then the likelihood of showing up and sticking with the commitment is slim to none.

Using a form will help you block off times that are available to you. First step is to block off times of any scheduled appointments. For example, if you work a traditional 9 to 5 schedule, then mid-morning and afternoon times may be out, which means early morning, lunchtime (possibly) and evening are IN! If you have any regularly scheduled evening meetings, block those off too.

When Will I Excersise?

	Sun	Mon	Tues	Wed	Thurs	Fri	Sat
Early Morning							
Mid-morning							
Lunchtime							
Afternoon							
Early Evening							
Evening							

www.staceycrewwellness.com

1. **Determine number of workouts per week**—If you haven't been doing any form of exercise, start with 30 minutes, 3 times per week. If you want to up what you're already doing, then commit to one additional workout per week.
2. **Consider your bio-rhythms.** What's the best time of day for you to excercise? This may be deteremined for you if you work during the day or have children home with you. But do your best to choose times that will work for you.
3. **Support**—Who is your support person and find a mutually good time for both of you.
4. **Plan**—Enter the workout times in the allotted slots.

Second step is to schedule the exercise time. If you haven't been exercising or moving, start small. Best to set a smaller goal of three times per week for twenty to thirty minutes and stick to it versus over-committing.

Note: a downloadable copy of the form is available at www. mindbodykitchenbook.com.

• Mindless vs. Mindful •

Mindless: Going about your day and NOT taking advantage of countless opportunities to move your body.

Mindful: Using every opportunity to move your body during the day by doing squats in between preparing coffee, getting up to refill your water bottle, or running laundry upstairs (or to another room) and putting it away.

CHAPTER 4

Nutrition 101

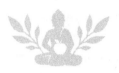

WHEN WE KNOW BETTER, we do better. Maya Angelou is most famous for saying it, and it's a quote I try to live by.

There are just a few simple strategies that you can put in place to quickly begin making better nutritional choices. This chapter introduces you to this simple but important nutrition information to understand how you can make simple, healthy choices every day, as well as some healthy options and substitutes.

Think of the last time you learned a new skill or took a class on a new topic. Once you learned the information, it became second nature, but there was an initial learning curve. Once you've mastered something though, you have the ability to move to the next level.

Nutrition works similarly by applying small changes over time that lead to some pretty big results. It does take some time, so give yourself the space to learn and grow. When I started improving what my family and I ate every day, I didn't have a lot of knowledge, but I was open to learning. So all I ask is that you do the same while experiencing some setbacks—because they happen! The key is to continue moving forward.

• Fueling Our Bodies •

Food is fuel. Give your body high-grade fuel to go the distance.

When it comes down to it, food is fuel for your body. Caring for our bodies with nutritious food is essential to improving and maintaining optimum performance. Healthy food makes our cells come alive and energizes us throughout the day. When I run and don't eat well, my mind and body suffer the consequences of too many calories burned and not enough nutrients to handle it.

You can liken your body to a vehicle that takes you through this life. In fact, imagine the most beautiful vehicle you've ever seen. What does it look like, how does it perform, where does it take you?

When you own an actual vehicle and you want it to last long after you've paid it off, you do several things to take care of it: change the oil, get routine tune-ups, and rotate the tires. If those routine maintenance tasks aren't done, then you wind up with a low-performing, gunky motor and bald tires, right?!

You also need to pump decent fuel into your car. If we continue to load our bodies with junk, our performance levels will drop and we'll become sluggish, tired, and weary.

Good news is that the converse is true: if we load our bodies with good, nutritious food, we can expect to function at a higher level with more energy to face the day and our lives.

Developing new habits and behaviors also requires time and thought to things like where we're hanging out—in this case, where we shop for food.

At the time I began improving what my family and I ate on a daily basis, I discovered that I actually didn't enjoy shopping at my local supermarket. And my kitchen wasn't set up to make simple, healthy meals. I had an overabundance of countertop appliances I didn't use that took up valuable countertop real estate.

My first challenge and goal was to upgrade what I was eating, so I focused on where to shop. The initial awareness had me choose another grocery store and I began shopping the perimeter of the store versus going up and down aisles, to avoid the processed food. I also learned how to read nutrition and ingredients labels, quickly realizing that many packaged foods contained an abundance of sodium—an inflammation-creating ingredient.

Did I mention it's a learning process?

I learned that sugar was another inflammation-provoking ingredient that provided absolutely no nutritional benefit. In fact, it was hurting way more than helping.

Furthermore, we've been trained to think that only protein comes from meat, which isn't true. You can actually get protein from many sources, including greens—spinach and broccoli, to name a couple. And eating organic and antibiotic-free meat is important. Otherwise we're ingesting whatever was injected into that animal while they were growing—this includes harmful chemicals—all of which can create inflammation in our bodies.

Today's food products (keyword is "products") offer little to no nutritional value. Packaged food is processed and processed food contains additives and additives give it shelf life but cause inflammation. This is a no-win situation for anyone attempting to improve their body's performance.

Processed, or manufactured, foods also contain high levels of sugar. When we eat too much sugar, it causes the body to have to work overtime. Add to that, if you're ingesting sugar and not exercising, the body will turn it into fat, which is stored and creates extra weight on the body.

A simple and solid goal is to strive for eating well 75% of the time to start, by making sure your staples (the food kept in your fridge and pantry) are healthy and learning to prepare and cook simple, healthy meals. This way, when you do go out to eat or to an event, you don't have to be ultra-concerned about the food that's being offered and you can more easily recover from ingesting high levels of sodium and sugar.

The interesting thing is that once you get used to eating real food, your taste buds and tummy will no longer tolerate unhealthy foods because they just don't taste good or make you feel good any longer.

It is necessary, however, to give your body an opportunity to embrace what it feels like to eat healthier. This is why my Three-Day Jumpstart (in the back of this book) or even the Whole30 are so effective. They are essentially elimination programs that remove all sugars and processed foods from your body, giving you an opportunity to "feel" how the body functions better when you nourish it with primarily plant-based, non-processed foods.

We also don't want to deprive ourselves but instead treat ourselves with grace and kindness. Deprivation only leads to setbacks and potential relapses. When things are off limits, it's natural to want those things—at heart, we're all just kids who want what we want.

Deprivation can also lead to giving up entirely or overeating. We also don't want to not eat. Yes, that's a double-negative. In simpler terms, we want to eat! We want to eat healthy foods that have our body's cells saying "Yay, I'm so happy I just want to dance!"

Thinking that no food is better than junk food can lead to the body shutting down and not functioning in a way that it needs to. Skipping meals will not help you slim down and if it does, the internal organs are NOT happy! Eventually, this will lead to problems that will take you straight to the doctor's office and into a cycle that in the end is much harder to manage.

Too much whine (and wine!) is not good either. Complaining and not taking responsibility for our own health and the way we eat will only lead to extra weight, lethargy, brain fog, fatigue, and lack of energy.

The body is a self-correcting organ. Oftentimes, simply giving it a balance of healthy food will restore it to normal working order. However, if you've been abusing your body for long periods of time by eating fast food on a regular basis, drinking too much alcohol, ingesting sugar daily—including cola—or depriving the body of food, it will take time to heal. But, IT IS possible.

The basic knowledge I'm about to teach you will help you move in the direction of making healthier choices and overall improvements in your health.

• Common Issues •

Over the years, I've discovered that many people make these common mistakes when it comes to their health:

- They lack basic knowledge.
- They don't get enough water.
- They don't eat enough greens.
- They lack a shopping strategy.
- They don't have enough time.
- They eat too many processed (boxed) foods.

Let's talk about each one and why these are important:

BASIC KNOWLEDGE

We make better decisions when we're armed with basic knowledge and tools. Throughout this book, you'll continue to learn how to simplify your decision-making process and upgrade your daily choices.

Back to the car maintenance analogy: We may not change the oil in our own car, but we do know that regular oil changes are incredibly important to the longevity of a car's engine. Well, with food it's similar. We may not understand how proteins are absorbed in the body or what fat to calories actually means, but if we know we need to reduce and/or eliminate sugar, drink more water, and eat more greens, a guaranteed byproduct is that the body will function at a higher level.

You don't have to have a degree in nutrition or biology. You simply need to incorporate simple, basic knowledge. This basic knowledge will do more to help you create a healthy diet and lifestyle than if you were to study an entire book about proteins, carbs, and calories.

In short, keep it simple, but take action!

NOT ENOUGH WATER

Did you know that most people are walking around dehydrated and don't even know it? Yup. The body is sixty percent water. As we go about our day, the water supply is depleted and we need to restore it. The 3:00 p.m. slump that has many looking to take a nap could actually be a result of dehydration. Instead of a cup of coffee or a soda, refill your water bottle and see if that revives you first.

Not all water is created equal.

The body performs best when it's in an alkaline state. Problem is, the American diet largely consists of acidic foods. Stay with me here and I'll explain. Meat is acidic, coffee is acidic, and anything with sugar creates acid in the body. When the body is in an acidic state, this creates a prime breeding ground for disease. In fact, diseases like cancer love an acidic environment and thrive on it. It's up to us to improve the body's interior by balancing it and creating an alkaline environment to ward off inflammation and disease.

That doesn't mean you need to avoid all of these foods and drinks but rather find balance and incorporate more alkaline food and liquids.

So back to water. Some waters are acidic in nature, and some tap water is better than bottled! An entire industry has been created around drinking water, but let's look at who's involved. The Coca-Cola Company "manufactures" and distributes Dasani water, which is one of the most acidic waters available on the market. They've managed to get into almost every sporting arena and vending machine. So, yes, we're "supposed" to drink more water, but unfortunately the water that's being provided is not only acidic but also addictive. Yup. Google it and read the ingredients label on the bottle. Dasani is not just water.

You also don't need expensive machines for your home. In fact, research this topic more on your own before making those decisions. Check your tap water by testing it with pH drops available on Amazon to see if it's better than bottled. And get yourself a reusable water bottle. Replace any carbonated and/or cola drinks with water and

I guarantee you'll have more energy and your body will thank you! Water also:

- Lubricates the body. Water provides the liquid necessary for us to digest our food. Little to no water can result in constipation and build up in the intestinal walls.

- Cleans out the liver. This is especially true with sugary foods and drinks, including alcohol. Without water, the liver will wind up storing sugar in the form of fat because it doesn't have any other way to move it through the system.

- Reduces inflammation. When we eat too much sodium and sugar (which are largely contained in processed foods) the body needs water to dilute sugar and sodium.

A simple way to determine whether your body is getting enough water is through your urine. Your pee should be clear. If it's yellow, cloudy, and has an odor, this is a sign that your body isn't hydrated, so start drinking—water, that is. If your urine is clear, you're likely on track with your daily hydration goals. Good job!

NOT ENOUGH GREENS

Many people also don't eat enough vegetables. In general, people tend to have an unfriendly relationship with vegetables. Whether it comes from not being encouraged to eat more veggies as a child or mainstream advertising pushing fast food, these messages are destroying our health.

More companies are promoting healthy foods, but corporate America still has a hold on mainstream TV commercials that are negatively impacting the choices most Americans make. Also, just because a food is labeled "natural" or "healthy" doesn't necessarily mean it is. These words have become commonplace for big food manufacturers to sell their foods to unsuspecting consumers. Always read the ingredients and nutritional facts labels.

Making a conscious effort to incorporate more vegetables into your daily diet can make all the difference. Greens contain vitamins and nutrients that will help your body run like the high-performance vehicle it is designed to be.

NO SHOPPING STRATEGY

In Chapter 6, "Meal Planning & Grocery Shopping," we'll discuss this in detail. It is, however, a very important part of why people lack healthy nutrition.

LACK OF TIME OR PREPARATION

In today's busy world, it can be hard to find time, but it's necessary for optimal health. This is also a form of self-care. Neglecting one's health has long-term, sometimes irreversible consequences. If it requires revamping schedules and tightening budgets, doing so is a preventative measure that allows life to be lived to the fullest.

TOO MANY PROCESSED FOODS

When we're relying on convenience foods or processed boxed foods, the body ultimately suffers. In order for food manufacturers to prolong the shelf life of boxed foods, they add chemicals, additives, and preservatives all of which create inflammation in the body and put it into an acidic state.

For the body to thrive, it needs whole foods that provide natural vitamins and minerals. Therefore, moving toward reducing, and eventually eliminating, processed foods is important to maintaining optimal health.

A good rule of thumb is to read the ingredients label and only choose a processed or boxed food IF it contains five or fewer ingredients and you recognize those ingredients without Googling them. Better choice is to eat more foods that don't contain a label.

• What You're Actually Eating •

It's not always possible to eat only foods without ingredients labels, such as fruits and vegetables, so here's some information about ingredients labels and the Recommended Dietary Allowance (RDA) that will help you make more informed decisions and understand exactly what you're choosing to eat.

• Recommended Dietary Allowance •

What we don't often take into consideration or realize is that the RDA that is listed on the ingredients label is based on a 2000-calorie per day diet. Problem is that when people's goals are to lose weight, they are typically aiming for fewer calories, so right away, this information is not entirely helpful.

Next we have Fat, Cholesterol, and Sodium. Note that the graphic below says to limit these, but what is the limit? I'll tell you! Again, based on a 2000-calorie per-day diet, here's the breakdown:

FAT: Forty-four grams. One avocado has between twenty and thirty grams of fat, of which about three grams are saturated fat. As a comparison, a Big Mac has twenty-nine grams of fat, but ten grams are saturated. Therefore, more than seventy-five percent of the fat in an avocado is "good fat," but in a Big Mac, more than fifty percent is "bad fat." So even though the total fat of an avocado and a Big Mac are not too different, the saturated fat in each of these foods creates the issue.

CHOLESTEROL: 300 milligrams maximum. The body needs cholesterol for hormone function and brain memory. Poor nutrition can lead to higher-than-recommended levels, which can require medication to reduce. Creating a healthy diet that includes more vegetables and foods low in saturated fats will help keep your cholesterol at a desired level for the body to function well.

SODIUM: 2,300 milligrams. If we're trying to drop a few pounds, we'll want to reduce that to about 1,800 immediately, and if we are prone to heart disease or high blood pressure (or over fifty years of age), that number should be reduced to about 1,100.

Next time you go to the grocery store, pick up a can of soup—any brand—and see what the sodium level is on the nutrition label. Also, check out the frozen dinners that have few calories—chances are they have higher levels of sodium and sugar.

Funny thing is, sugar is not highlighted on this label example below. My feeling is that although there's talk about sugar, it still hasn't been outed as the highly addictive ingredient it is.

Nutrition Facts

8 servings per container
Serving size 2/3 cup (55g)

Amount per serving
Calories 230

	% Daily Value*
Total Fat 8g	**10%**
Saturated Fat 1g	**5%**
Trans Fat 0g	
Cholesterol 0mg	**0%**
Sodium 160mg	**7%**
Total Carbohydrate 37g	**13%**
Dietary Fiber 4g	**14%**
Total Sugars 12g	
Includes 10g Added Sugars	**20%**
Protein 3g	
Vitamin D 2mcg	10%
Calcium 260mg	20%
Iron 8mg	45%
Potassium 240mg	6%

* The % Daily Value (DV) tells you how much a nutrient in a serving of food contributes to a daily diet. 2,000 calories a day is used for general nutrition advice.

Figure 1: U.S. Food and Drug Administration

Don't forget to read the actual ingredients. This is the list of everything that has been used to make the processed foods. Instead of asking yourself, "Is it okay for me to eat?" ask instead, "Do I really want to eat Yellow #5, or any chemical for that matter? Will my body thank me for it?"

The famous Kraft Macaroni and Cheese Dinner ingredients include many that aren't and easily identifiable. My favorite is "cheese sauce mix." So there is no real cheese in this product?!

SERVING SIZE

Pay close attention to the serving size on food boxes, too. When you pick up a boxed food from the grocery store, check the serving size. Chances are, it won't feel like enough because when we go out to eat, the portion sizes are typically quite large.

Kraft Macaroni and Cheese has a serving size of 2.5 ounces, which equates to ⅓ cup. And the sodium level in a serving is 660 mg. Is that really worth the inflammation it's going to cause in your body? Why not make a healthier version that includes whole grain pasta and nutritional yeast—real ingredients.

To avoid potentially harmful ingredients, steer clear of the following:

- Anything that ends in "ose." This is a clue that it contains a form of sugar. This includes the famed "high fructose corn syrup," which is a big cause of inflammation.
- Xanthan gum. This is a thickening agent that's used to "hold" ingredients together.
- Anything that starts with "Yellow Number . . . " This is a chemical dye used to create a particular color in food.
- Low-fat. This means that it's likely loaded with chemicals to compensate for the lack of fat.
- Low-sodium. Again, loaded with preservatives like sugar.

SUGAR

For years, I was an almost daily Dunkin Donuts drive-through customer, ordering the regular: a Boston cream donut and a large, iced coffee. This started around the time my daughters were preschoolers. My go-to method to get my oldest to take a nap was to drive her around in the car, so I would roll through the drive-thru once she was asleep and munch down the donut and sip on the large, iced coffee before we arrived home and I was able to transfer her inside.

I rationalized this as my well-deserved treat for being a hard-working mama. No doubt I was a hard-working mama, but my attitude about how I rewarded myself came from a place of not understanding the negative effects this routine was having on my mind and body. Looking back on it, I never felt good after this routine. My body never "thanked" me. Instead, I would crash and feel even worse once the sugar wore off. I'm certain too that although I didn't experience any external weight gain, I was most certainly walking around with a body that was—to use the car analogy—low on oil, needing a tune-up and almost out of gas.

Sugar is addictive. Studies show that it's as addictive as street drugs, and it's everywhere. We've become a "dessert for breakfast" society where we launch our day with empty calories and a sugar rush. That quickly leads to the next fix or a crash that affects not only our mood but our productivity levels.

Soda is the worst! The daily recommended value of sugar each day is six teaspoons. A twelve-ounce soda (not sixteen) contains nine teaspoons of sugar. One can and you're already over the daily budget.

Sugar cravings are real, too. Once you eat a little, your body craves more. It can become a never-ending obsession. And if you know anything about addiction, it's really hard to maintain normal relationships when your primary goal each day is to satisfy a sugar craving. Okay, so maybe that's a little extreme, but not too far off the mark because sugar addiction wreaks havoc on your mind and body.

At one point, I did switch my sugar addiction to a daily venti

Caramel Macchiato from Starbucks, cutting out the donut, but the amount of sugar in one of those babies is thirty-three grams, or just more than six and a half teaspoons. Again, over the limit!

It's important to understand that our U.S. system of communicating measurements is confusing. The fact that ingredients labels measure in grams and RDA measure in teaspoons has most people either guessing or giving up when it comes to figuring out what they're actually eating. The general public thinks that the government and food manufacturers have our backs, but they don't. They are in the business of selling food products.

Gradually I cut out big sugary drinks and adopted a healthy breakfast that includes protein and natural sugars, such as strawberries and blueberries.

It takes time to acclimate to eating non-processed foods if this has been our primary food source. For optimal health, it's important that we work toward making healthier choices. It's a proactive measure that, in the long run, is easier than dealing with the health issues that result when we don't pay attention. It's up to us to take responsibility for our health.

In order to make changes, we must first acknowledge our current behaviors, patterns, and habits. This food journal exercise will help you make the connection between what you eat and how it makes you feel.

• Exercise 1: Five Days of Food Journaling •

We must understand our existing behaviors and habits before we can really know what we need to change. The best way to make a healthy shift in our food choices starts with understanding what happens to our bodies and minds when we eat certain foods.

This is no easy feat, but it is important. The good news is you don't have to make any changes in what you're eating right now. You just need to record what you're eating and how these foods make you feel. Then you'll be able to identify the shifts that need to occur and move to creating the ideal diet for YOU!

Record what you eat (all meals, snacks, drinks, condiments, etc.) for at least five days. It's important that you also record the times you ate. More important is recording how you felt after eating specific foods. When you get in touch with how food makes you feel, then you can make better decisions about the healthiest foods for YOUR body.

Ready, set, GO!

DAY ONE

TIME: _____

BREAKFAST:_____

What did you notice about the choice you made to eat?

_____

For example, was it the "usual" or the only thing in the fridge or pantry? Did you not feel like preparing breakfast? Whatever it is, write it!

How I felt after eating: _____

_____

For example: satisfied, still hungry, lethargic, energized, bloated. Also list any of the following:

Physical feedback, such as bloating, headache, fatigue, insomnia, energy, or satisfaction.
Emotional feedback such as irritated, anxious, lethargic, calm, or joyful.

TIME: _____

SNACK: _____

How I felt after eating: _____
What did you notice about the choice you made to eat?

_____

TIME: _____

LUNCH: _____

What did you notice about the choice you made to eat?

_____

How I felt after eating: _____

TIME: _____

DINNER: _____

What did you notice about the choice you made to eat?

_____

How I felt after eating: _____

TIME: _____

OTHER: _____

What did you notice about the choice you made to eat?

_____

How I felt after eating: _____

Once you've worked through Five Days of Food Journaling, then return and work through the exercise below to create a new habit, which will involve incorporating what you learned in the food journal exercise.

But keep reading! You want to continue learning and incorporating what's contained in this book to maintain momentum and create momentum toward change and a healthier lifestyle.

• Exercise 2: Creating a New Habit •

Creating change doesn't come without some work, but IT IS possible with a little focus and commitment.

Since you're reading this book, it's safe to say that you are committed to making changes and improving your overall health and wellness.

Over the years, I've used many techniques to incorporate new habits. Everything from restricting myself from certain activities so I wouldn't be tempted to eat sweets, or accountability to a friend or coach to keep me on task with my exercise routine.

The accountability factor works! That's why we will use a combination of this exercise, followed by accountability in the Facebook group (www.facebook.com/groups/mindbodykitchen) created specifically for this program.

Ready, set, GO!

1. First, let's identify what habits you've tried to create in the past and why they haven't worked. List below five habits you've attempted to create in the past. This could be anything from no more nail biting to exercising regularly to limiting daily complaints.

    a.

    b.

    c.

    d.

    e.

When you think about why each one hasn't worked, begin to analyze the roadblocks preventing the habit from sticking. Ask yourself questions such as: Was the time of day you chose to exercise not working? Did you just not feel like moving? Was confusion about what to buy or frustration with the shopping process the reason you only had unhealthy snack options during your last healthy eating attempt?

2. List five habits/behaviors you'd like to develop:

   a.

   b.

   c.

   d.

   e.

3. Return to the list above and cross off any habits listed that you would NOT change for yourself. Since changing for other people doesn't generally work, let's focus on something you want to do for yourself.

4. Choose one habit/behavior from the remaining items and enter it below:

   _____

   This will be your focus.

5. Are there any barriers to changing this habit/behavior? If the answer is yes, what are those barriers?

   _____

   _____

   _____

   _____

   _____

6. Is this still a realistic choice of behavior to change? Yes / No If no, redo numbers four and five. If yes, proceed to step seven.

7. Take out your calendar, review the week's upcoming activities and commitments, and enter time on the calendar to devote to working on your new habit.

Block out at least three to four fifteen-minute slots each week to devote to changing this behavior. If you can do more, do more, but be realistic. Best to strive for small successes, then add to it! How you spend your time changing this habit is up to you. I encourage you to come over to the Facebook group and share your commitment and ask for support and suggestions on how to make this change, if needed. But please don't get into the weeds on asking for suggestions. It's more important to create the new habit than talk about it.

ACTION IS ESSENTIAL!

• Exercise 3: Creating Your Ideal Diet •

Diet is a tricky word. When most people hear the word diet, they think of a regimented food plan of things that don't taste good or they really don't want to eat. So, typically, a diet is a negative experience!

My definition of "diet" is what you choose to eat each day, which has no restrictions. You're here to learn how to eat healthier, so let's talk about a "healthy diet," which still doesn't need restrictions.

What if you could create a daily "diet" of foods you love that also nourishes your body?

Let's do it!

Here's where we shift your perspective and create the ideal diet for YOU.

1. Before reading this book, what did the word "diet" mean to you? (Use another piece of paper if you feel compelled to go deep here. This could mean writing about your early experiences as an adolescent, teenager, or young woman. I encourage you to take the time to delve into this and discover more about yourself and your relationship to food.)

_____

_____

_____

_____

_____

2. What feelings and emotions surround the word diet? Does it bring about a sense of accomplishment or failure? Enthusiasm or dread?

_____

_____

_____

_____

_____

3. What diets have you tried in the past and what were the results?

_____

_____

_____

_____

_____

4. Based on what you learned, which foods do you know taste good and make your body feel good? How do they make you feel?

_____

_____

_____

_____

_____

5. Based on what you learned about sugar, estimate how much sugar you eat each day. Remember, this could be in the form of a soda drink, a donut, processed foods, etc.

_____

_____

_____

6. How can you adjust your daily choices so you're putting healthier food into your daily diet?

Breakfast:

_____

_____

Lunch:

_____

_____

Dinner:

_____

_____

Snacks:

_____

_____

Drinks:

_____

_____

Now that you have the information above, how can you challenge yourself to create food choices that do not contain processed food? Which meals can you prepare to put you on a healthier path?

Use the Three-Day Jump Start as a jumping off point to make healthier choices and create a custom "diet" for YOU.

_____

_____

_____

_____

_____

• Mindless vs. Mindful •

MINDLESS: Dumping loads of sugar and processed foods into your body, creating an unhealthy gut, foggy brain, and a breeding ground for disease.

MINDFUL: Providing your body with the nutrients it needs to run like a high-performance car.

Armed with knowledge of self and nutrition, we're now going to learn how to create a kitchen you love.

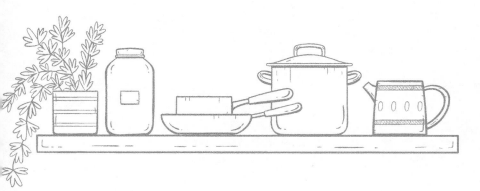

Part Two

CREATING A HEALTHY KITCHEN

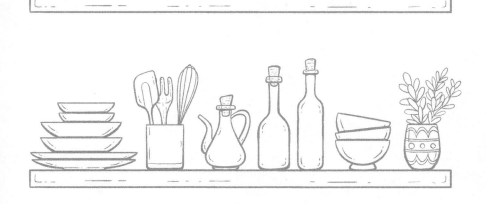

CHAPTER 5

A Precursor to Organizing
Your Kitchen: What to Consider

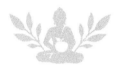

• What Is a Healthy Kitchen? •

A healthy kitchen is clean, organized, and open for business.

A healthy kitchen is also stocked with fresh and healthy ingredients. However, there are other things to consider. This chapter guides you through the steps to create a healthy kitchen, which includes the introduction of concepts to help you see your kitchen from a different perspective; how to zone it for maximum efficiency; and how to overcome decision fatigue that can keep you from creating a kitchen you love.

The kitchen has always been one of my favorite rooms of the home. Even after the Broccoli Incident, I still loved the kitchen. It truly is the heart of the home because it's where we nourish ourselves and our family. However, for most of my adult life, I did not enjoy grocery shopping at all. I would approach it as a "stocking up" recon mission vs. a "planning to nourish myself and my family" task. I dashed in and grabbed what I could without making any real sense of how it would all come together, then dashed out.

I'd fill plastic bags with fruit that would make a pretty centerpiece and get boxes of frozen dinners that would nicely line the inside of the freezer. More than once, I bought a collection of cheeses I stacked neatly in the fridge. It looked more like I was planning a party than creating simple, healthy meals.

My priorities were a little off. I was shopping to make things look nice rather than considering what ingredients I liked, or actually needed, in order to prepare a meal.

The process wasn't fun, and I basically just wanted to get in and out of the store, get home and make it look like we were prepared for the week. I was also spending an extraordinary amount of money, not realizing that shopping healthier could actually save me money, too.

• Grocery Shopping •

Grocery stores don't always stock the shelves with nourishing foods and ingredients. That, combined with the onslaught of advertisements from big food manufacturers, leaves many people choosing low-quality food "products" that are loaded with chemicals. And as I mentioned in Chapter 4, many processed foods today contain addictive ingredients that never satiate, but instead leave us wanting for more and more of the same addictive foods.

As a certified health coach, one of the first recommendations I make to clients is this: If you want to eat healthier, then buy healthier food; don't bring foods into your home that are unhealthy or that will tempt you. This is easier said than done, but it's a habit that can be developed over time.

When you're making changes in habits and routines, sometimes it's necessary to change locations, too. In this case, it can mean changing where you shop. Going to the most convenient grocery store may not give you the ingredients and choices you need to begin to eat and cook healthier food.

During my efforts to eat healthier, I was repeatedly annoyed with the grocery shopping process. After analyzing why I was frustrated,

I determined that it was important for me to have better options, lower prices, and fewer choices to avoid decision fatigue, which we will discuss later in this chapter. I also realized that the most convenient grocery store to my home didn't meet any of the criteria. In fact, the section labeled "Health Food" was literally eight feet of freezer space, leaving me to wonder whether the rest of the food in the store was unhealthy.

Each time I shopped at this grocery store, I was never completely satisfied. I would haul the packages home, unload items into the fridge and pantry, and then ask myself, "What's for dinner?" Frequently, I'd pick up the phone and order a pizza because there was no actual plan.

After researching the grocery stores in my city, I ended up choosing a store thirty minutes from my home, but it became a pleasant process. On the drive there and back, I could listen to a favorite podcast, then breeze in and out of the store relatively quickly, get healthier ingredients and food options, and feed my family foods that were nourishing and delicious.

Thanks to my new strategy, I actually began to enjoy shopping. I cooked and ate the items I brought home because the quality was better and I was satisfied with the price points, too. My grocery store of choice became one of my happy places.

So when it comes to where you shop, ask yourself the following questions:

1. Am I satisfied with the options at my grocery store? Yes/No
2. Does my grocery store have too many options that makes it overwhelming? Yes/No
3. Do I feel like I get good quality for the price? Yes/No
4. Does the store provide products with high-quality ingredients? Yes/No
5. When I bring home my grocery haul, am I excited about what I'm going to prepare? Yes/No

Note: in Chapter 6, "Meal Planning & Grocery Shopping," there's an exercise for shopping strategies to make this process more tolerable, if not enjoyable.

• Overcome Decision Fatigue and Simplify •

It may seem a little odd to introduce the idea of decision fatigue in a chapter about a healthy kitchen, but here's why: during the day, we make lots and lots of decisions—what to wear, which tasks to focus on to meet work goals, how the kids will get to their activities and who will drive them, etc.

On top of everything else that needs to get done, add in learning how to make healthier choices. With all of this, the brain can become fatigued; by the time dinner rolls around, you feel done for the day and unprepared to make the best decisions about dinner. As a result, you have no desire to cook a healthy meal.

We're also talking about this before we move on to how to organize and zone the kitchen so you're armed with the power to make good shopping decisions—so you can get the results you seek.

• Decision Making •

I also want to highlight the idea of indecision and how this can keep us stuck when it comes to making change. This comes from many years working as a professional organizer and understanding how clutter oftentimes is a result of indecision. I've learned that the biggest reason people get stuck and avoid making decisions is fear of making the wrong one. However, not making a decision will never keep you moving forward, but only keep you stuck. Even if the decision you make is ultimately not the right one, at you least made one.

When people ask how long it takes to declutter and organize anything, my question is always: "how quickly can you make decisions?"

To make a decision, first you need to consider the space, activity or situation. Next, get clear on what you want the outcome to look like. Then determine the criteria for making the decision. And finally, start deciding!

Making decisions will lead you toward the final result. So start deciding and if it's not the right decision in the moment, congratulate yourself for making progress, then move on to making another decision.

When it comes to kitchen clutter, you might use the following criteria: (1) if I haven't used it in six months, then it goes, or (2) if it has a chip in it or it's broken and I don't want to expend the energy to fix or have it fixed, then it goes.

Here are some easy ways to approach decisions when it comes to pantry and fridge items:

1. You have pantry items that haven't been used in six months. Question: will you eat them? Probably not, so that's a donation to a food bank. Great job, you've just made a decision!

2. If it no longer fits with our new way of eating—for example, you've chosen to not eat anything that contains ingredients you can't pronounce—then decide to toss it. You just made another decision. Woohoo! You're on a roll.

3. You've chosen to eat only organic and you have canned foods that are still in date. You decide to donate to a local food bank. Done, decision. Pat yourself on the back.

4. In the pantry, you have a serving platter that is broken, so you decide to toss it. One less thing to manage that you weren't using. Keep going!

5. In the refrigerator, you have condiments that have surpassed their expiration date, so you toss. Awesome!

I've included a list on how to set criteria when purging items from your pantry and fridge in the exercises at the end of this chapter. Just remember: movement forward requires decision making, so start brushing up on your skills.

Let me reiterate: the amount of time it takes to organize depends on two things:

(1) How much stuff you have and (2) How quickly you can make decisions.

So if you have a fridge or a pantry that hasn't been organized in a long time or is jam-packed with all sorts of stuff, you'll need to adjust your estimate of how long it will take based on your personal pacing.

• Reduce Decision Fatigue •

Think of your favorite restaurant specials. We all have that one restaurant we can count on to consistently deliver a delicious meal that meets expectations every time. Why? Because they've perfected it! And you can too. This will reduce the decisions you have to make and simplify the process by creating a repertoire of healthy meals that work.

If you don't already have your "specialty dish," then choose something you love and work to make it your signature dish, perfecting it over time. Then add another dish. And another. Eventually, you create a bank of meals that you no longer need the recipes for because you can make it from memory—and they're delicious. If your current signature dish contains ingredients that aren't supporting your efforts to eat healthier, challenge yourself to upgrade the ingredients, creating a healthier version of a dish you love.

Don't worry about others getting tired of the same dishes. The goal here is to create a SYSTEM to save you time, energy and money. Teach family members how to cook too, and if they don't like something, challenge them to come up with a meal that they can perfect. Cooking is a skill that everyone should have—and I don't use the word "should" lightly here. Kids especially need this skill so they can take care of themselves as adults. If you do have children, involve them and learn together.

• Not Organizing for Your Current Lifestyle •

Every time I've finished an organizing job, we'd end up with extra containers. Why? Because once clients became clear on their "why," it became very apparent that much of what they thought was important no longer served them. Out the door it went.

This was the case with Jackie and Mark who had a pantry stocked to the gills. Mark loved to barbecue, so anytime they were out shopping or traveling and he stumbled across something barbecue-related, such as sauces or utensils, he would buy it and place it in the pantry. Mark was so proud of his collection that he couldn't wait to show-and-tell his guests about his barbecuing paraphernalia conquests.

There was just one problem. They lived in an apartment that prohibited barbecues on the balcony. So the collection kept growing but never got used. These items would work for their future home but didn't suit their current lifestyle. It took up valuable real estate they could've used for their current needs.

We talked about their goal date for buying a house. I recommended that if it wasn't in the next six months, and we couldn't find some unused storage space in the home, they should consider boxing it up and storing it at their in-laws home until they had a home—and a barbecue!

As we progressed with their kitchen organization, they also determined that barbecuing wasn't the healthiest way to prepare meat. Mark was trying to reduce inflammation in his body and the ingredients did not align with his health goals. Some bottles of sauces contained a lot of sugar and sodium. Although Mark resisted this information initially, his overall goal was to lose weight and improve his overall health.

Too often people are not living in alignment with the lifestyle they actually desire or didn't realize they deserved. Either they are focused on "when" or what used to be instead of embracing the reality of their current situation and how it affects their health.

Mark ultimately decided to give his barbecue collection to a friend with a backyard. That way, he could still periodically enjoy one of his favorite meals with friends, while freeing up space in his pantry and focusing on making healthier daily choices.

• Healthy Kitchen Guidelines •

Health is more than what we put into our bodies. It's our surroundings, how we think, who we hang out with, and how we feel when we're engaged in a particular activity. By asking yourself "does this feel good?"—especially in the kitchen—and tapping into the five senses, you'll begin to make this space healthier.

First, let's define (by now, you know I love to do this for you) the terms *cleaning* and *organizing*, which are important for this chapter and the remainder of the book.

Cleaning is defined as the act of making something free of dirt, marks, or mess, especially by washing, wiping, or brushing.

Organizing is the act of arranging things into a structured order OR into a structured or whole.

So often, I hear people describe how they've been "cleaning" all day when they haven't even taken out the vacuum or dust cloth yet. What they've actually been doing is organizing. And when things are organized, cleaning takes less time and is so much easier.

While it's important to separate these two tasks, sometimes you'll do both at the same time. However, by focusing on decluttering and organizing your kitchen, eliminating unnecessary counter clutter, and removing or storing things you don't use regularly elsewhere, you will create an environment in which you can create a healthy meal and clean up quickly.

A healthy kitchen is:

1. Clean. The last thing we want to do before preparing a meal is clean the kitchen. We need clean surfaces and an empty sink to begin so we don't run into obstacles. To

maintain a clean kitchen, clean up after each meal, which includes emptying the sink by filling the dishwasher, taking out the trash, and wiping down the countertops. Of course, I also recommend a deeper cleaning once a week.

2. Organized. When things are organized effectively, meaning relevant and within reach, we can quickly accomplish the tasks at hand. Think about a time when you've stayed in an Airbnb or a vacation rental. Typically, everything is organized and set up so you can easily find what you need when you need it. Same goes for your home.

3. Open for business. When the kitchen is "open" (remember to set the open hours and, more importantly, closed hours, to avoid mindless snacking so you stay focused on your wellness goals), anyone can quickly and easily make something healthy to eat. Think about guests—could they easily find what they need?

4. Stocked with healthy ingredients. After reading Chapter 4 called "Nutrition 101," consider upgrading your ingredients. Read the labels and replace (either by using or donating) what you have with healthier options. If you don't bring junk food into the home, you'll be less likely to eat it, so fill your fridge and pantry with options that positively contribute to a healthy mind and body.

5. Uncluttered. Eliminating counter clutter creates more workspace and makes cleaning the countertops easier. Regain space in the kitchen by removing anything that doesn't relate to food and creating, simple healthy meals.

6. Well lit. Consider the lighting and explore ways to shed brighter light on your kitchen workspaces. A friend of mine who works as a personal chef shared how upgraded

lighting in a client's kitchen changed everything. The client eventually wound up spending more time in the space creating healthy, home-cooked meals on his own.

• Exercise 1: Finding Your Why •

How many of us embark on a new adventure or change in our lives without the preparation truly needed to set ourselves up for success?

Imagine you've hit the road for a cross-country trip on the spur of the moment. You get fifty miles down the road and realize you've forgotten your favorite sunglasses, or worse, your glasses that you need for night driving. You haven't made hotel arrangements in advance and don't have much cash. You're basically unprepared.

Then imagine that you've taken time to plan your trip. You've researched hotels, found some deals, planned how much cash you'll need, packed snacks/food, your favorite pillow, and checked off other items on your list. You get on the road, you're relaxed and feeling positive about your adventure.

Understanding your why is a great predictor of how successful you'll be on your journey. In order to define your *why*, you'll want to outline your goals first. For example, if your goal is to lose weight, but you don't identify how many pounds you want to lose, then there's no real goal to aim for. Likewise, if your goal is to improve your sleep but you lack specifics (eight hours of uninterrupted sleep, for example) and don't prepare, you have no real target to understand whether you've reached your goal.

So when it comes to a healthier lifestyle, think about what you'd like to achieve in the end. Consider the new habits you'll need to develop so the process of creating this new lifestyle sticks. The sooner you discover these pieces, the sooner you'll understand that change is a process. Defining your why is the key to success. It's like planning out a trip; even if you have detours along the way, you're still headed toward the final destination. To define your why, asking yourself the following questions:

1. What do you consider your biggest challenge?
2. What is motivating you currently?
3. What do you intend to accomplish?
4. What is your goal?
5. What will your life look like once you've reached your goal?

Spend some time on this. Grab a notebook or journal and free write, then re-read and create a three to five sentence statement of your goal, clearly defining the results you seek. Here's an example of a why statement:

My why is to help create a healthy lifestyle that will contribute positively to my future. Specifically, I want to eat mindfully each day to lose fifteen pounds. I will also move my body at least four times a week for thirty minutes and aim for seven to eight hours of sleep each night. All of this will push me to be the best version of myself so that I can live a long and happy life with my family and friends.

KITCHEN VISION

Once you've created your why statement, decide how you'd like your kitchen to look and feel. Peruse Pinterest and look at kitchen examples for inspiration. Chances are, what you see online will have clear counters and be functional versus full of tchotchkes and counter clutter. It doesn't matter if you're a visual person or a minimalist or someone who likes to collect things.

The kitchen is the room where you nourish yourself and your family, so you want to keep distractions to a minimum to allow you to focus on the important task, which is creating healthy meals.

You want to be able step into the kitchen and do the following easily and smoothly:

- Choose what you'll make.

- Easily locate the tools you need.
- Serve the meal.
- Clean up.
- Leave.

The ability to leave is important when you're trying to remain healthy. Too many people hang out in the kitchen. And when you hang out in the kitchen, you wind up snacking. Like a restaurant, set hours of operation and "close" the kitchen.

This is one of the healthiest things you can do for you and your family.

Health comes in various forms and stages. The word *healthy* has many meanings, depending upon the context. In terms of someone's physical health, healthy means free of disease or pain. In terms of emotional well-being, you could say that someone has a healthy appetite. Then there's the use of the word in terms of food, which means free from contamination or toxins. A healthy kitchen is one that is clean, organized, and open for business.

• Three Elements of a Healthy Kitchen •

Now let's talk about each of the three elements of a healthy kitchen so you can make it a reality in your own home:

Organized. You can easily find what you need, when you need it!

How often do we attempt to cook something and realize we need to empty the dishwasher first, then load the dishwasher with the dishes that were left in the sink? Or maybe we need to empty the trash because we don't have enough space to put scraps from the vegetables we're about to peel?

Healthy ingredients. The fridge contains fresh food and ingredients to create a simple and healthy meal.

How often do we go to cook something, haven't planned, and don't have the one ingredient on hand that makes all the difference?

We either scrap the cooking and call for takeout or get in the car and buy the ingredients to finish the meal-in-progress.

Tools. You have the right tools for the right jobs. And you'd be surprised how few tools you actually need to create most meals.

As a professional organizer, I spent many years helping individuals declutter and organize their homes. I've been in many kitchens where families struggled to prepare meals, mainly due to the clutter, especially on the countertops. Because we can all use a little decluttering, it's important for me to bring you a tried-and-proven organizing method: For one week, each time you use a kitchen tool (including pots and pans), leave it out on the counter after washing it. At the end of the week, see what you've used. Most likely, it's the same five to seven tools.

Let's run through a few of the major issues that create kitchen clutter:

1. Too many items in the kitchen. The kitchen hasn't been decluttered and could use some purging.
2. Cabinets full of unused items. This may include collections of coffee mugs and plastic cups from events. It also may include unopened ketchup packets and chopsticks, along with a barrage of things that live in the space but may have a better home outside the kitchen.
3. Countertops used for storage. This happens when the cabinets are cluttered with unused items—or perhaps too many items—or things simply aren't put away. Rearranging items in appropriate zones will help create optimum organization.

• Problem? Solved! •

Once I worked with a family that had an extreme situation. They had a kitchen where not only were the cabinets full of items, but the stovetop and the countertops were too, making it impossible to cook or prepare food. The family had even gone as far as buying extra shelving units and placing them in the eating area of the kitchen to house even more stuff.

First, we created a purging area that included donate boxes. Although you would think it would make sense to begin with the obvious clutter we could see on the countertops and shelving, instead, we focused on what was in the closed cabinets. They were packed with unused items because what was being used lived on the countertops and shelving.

By clearing these items, we were then able to focus on the countertops and shelving clutter, purging what was no longer needed and placing the remainder in the cabinets, ultimately clearing the countertops, which made room for food preparation.

It became apparent that we needed to have a conversation about how much space they actually had to store items versus the amount of stuff they had. The client confessed to being a garage sale shopper who bought items because they were a good deal even though she had no place to put them. She also fell victim to the countless advertisements that came in the mail for countertop appliances, knowing deep down that she didn't need them, but struggling to turn down a deal.

The thing is, the price may be good, but nothing is a good deal if you don't use it or truly have no space to store it. Because they had too many items for the kitchen, I recommended they keep only what they would use on a regular basis, which ultimately allowed them to clear the countertops and eliminate the shelving. These two things moved them toward creating a healthy kitchen: one that was clean, organized, and open for business!

I also coached the client on shifting her Saturday morning garage sale routine to something that didn't cost any money, like walking in the park, and an activity that also didn't involve acquiring "new" items. It took a little effort, but by making those shifts, her kitchen stayed uncluttered, she was able to prepare healthy meals, AND she wound up dropping fifteen pounds because she was consistently moving her body.

• Zoning the Kitchen •

Zoning the kitchen is the first step in creating a healthy kitchen.

Zones create specific areas for specific activities and have distinctive features and characteristics that separate them from the other zones. They also divide space into usable sections and provide direction on where to store items for a particular task. Bottom line is that it's easier to understand how a particular room functions when there are clear zones.

Kindergarten and Montessori classrooms are notorious for this type of set up, making it easy for children to understand what happens in a particular area of the room. It also helps when it's time to clean up because everything has a specific home.

Zones also help you to decide where to place items. For example, in a kitchen, you would place dishes in the "Serving" zone and sponges in the "Cleaning/Dishwashing" zone. It may sound remedial or elementary to talk about zoning your rooms like a kindergarten classroom, but the key to organizing, and making things efficient, is to make them as uncomplicated as possible.

For overall kitchen organization, you'll want to divide and conquer. Typically, most kitchens are designed with the traditional "work triangle" in mind. A work triangle is an uninterrupted traffic pattern where the stove, sink, and refrigerator are positioned on different sides of a triangular pattern, usually no more than nine feet apart. For purposes of this organization book, we will assume that your kitchen has the traditional work triangle. (But please don't let this bog you down if it doesn't. Once you are organized, it won't really matter.)

Now let's now divide and conquer using five zones in your kitchen:

1. Food preparation
2. Cooking
3. Cleaning
4. Serving
5. Food storage

You may want to add additional zones such as arts and crafts—if you have a large kitchen where small children gather to color or do crafts—or a family communication zone where you house the family calendar. But let's focus on the five primary zones first!

First we'll do a run-through on how this works and then follow that with a specific exercise you can implement in your own kitchen. Note: you can use zoning in any room of your home and I encourage you to do so. For now, we'll focus on the kitchen.

• How It Works •

You'll want to start by identifying and assigning areas within the kitchen for specific activities. You may already have a nicely organized kitchen, but there's always room for improvement, so I would encourage you to do this exercise. Looking at something with a fresh set of eyes can help you tweak what you already have in place, making it even more efficient. For example, maybe you keep the spices in the pantry, which is located across the room from the stove where you use spices, and now you realize that they might be better located in the cabinets above the stove.

This exercise is also meant to help you consciously think about how to make your life easier in the kitchen. So take your time and use this as an opportunity to simplify and make your space more efficient.

FIVE RECOMMENDED ZONES

These are the five main kitchen zones and what you need to know about each one:

Food Preparation Zone

Where to put it: Near the sink, if possible
What to store here: Mixing bowls, measuring cups, wooden spoons, knives, cutting board, and miscellaneous appliances (mixer, chopper, blender)

Tip: Keep a good-quality cutting board nearby and keep knives sharpened to make food prep easier.

Cooking/Baking Zone

Where to put it: Near the stove
What to store here: Spices, pots and pans, and utensils
Tip: Maintain the freshness of your baking supplies and avoid pesky critters by placing flour, sugar, and so on in sealed, labeled containers. Mason jars work well. They are available online or at the grocery store (in some areas) and are an inexpensive and easily-accessible option.

Serving Zone

Where to put it: Near the kitchen table or eating area
What to store here: Serving dishes, plates, bowls, glassware, utensils, and napkins
Tip: If you're cramped for cabinet space but have room near the kitchen table, consider adding a sideboard or buffet to house dishes, plates, and bowls. That makes for easy access when setting the table for a meal. If you tend to plate food at the counter area, locate plates, dishes, and bowls in a cabinet close to the stove.

Cleaning/Dishwashing Zone

Where to put it: Near the sink or dishwasher
What to store here: Soap, sponges, and brushes
Tip: If possible, store cleaning supplies in an overhead cabinet to avoid little ones gaining access. To avoid dishpan hands, wear rubber gloves when cleaning pots and pans. Keep hand lotion nearby.

Food Storage Zone

Where to put it: Near the refrigerator
What to store here: Containers for leftovers, along with plastic wrap and tinfoil.

Tip: When you're storing leftovers, use containers that you can record the date you store it. Organize them with the oldest at the front in a designated area in the fridge. Work them into your meal plan within a few days.

• Exercise 1: Zoning the Kitchen •

Follow these steps to clearly identify the work triangle and the zones within your kitchen space. Once you've done that, relocate what is currently outside of a zone into the newly-designated zones.

1. Draw a rough layout of your kitchen as if you were looking down on it from above. DO NOT stress over making it perfect. This is not an art project.

2. Identify the work triangle by creating dotted lines between the stove, refrigerator and sink.

3. Identify the five zones in your kitchen space by using different colors; draw a circle or square (whichever is more appropriate given the space) around the zone. Note: some zones may overlap and that's okay.

    a. Food preparation
    b. Cooking
    c. Cleaning
    d. Serving
    e. Food Storage

4. Once you have identified the zones, put all related items in the appropriate zones. This may require reorganizing cabinets.

Other considerations

Group like things together. For instance, if you're a coffee drinker, set up a coffee station that includes the coffee pot, coffee mugs, creamer, sugar bowl, and spoon. Further, to keep it simple, put the coffee pot next to the sink so you can easily fill the pot with water.

Add additional zones. These may include a beverage/snack station, a family communication center (see Resources section). If you have a baby or small children, consider a zone for items such as bottles, baby food, or sippy cups. If you have toddlers, preschoolers, or elementary-age children, consider incorporating an arts and crafts zone to store paper, crayons, washable markers, and coloring books so your little one can entertain themself while you're preparing a meal.

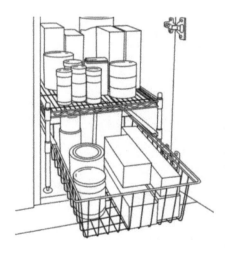

Incorporate baskets. If you're not in a position to install semi-custom or custom pull-out drawers to make lower cabinets easier to access, use baskets that you can easily access for pot lids and other small items. Use one basket per category.

Keep countertops uncluttered.

Countertops are valuable real estate in the kitchen, so use this space wisely. If you're not using an appliance on a daily basis, you may want to consider placing it in a cabinet, leaving more room for food preparation. Consider purging items in the cabinets to make room or relocate non-kitchen items to another part of the house. For example, put paperwork in the office or projects in closed storage in the family room.

• Mindless vs. Mindful •

Mindless: Continuing to use your kitchen in the same way you always have, not making tweaks and expecting different results.

Mindful: Using a set of fresh eyes and making tweaks in the kitchen so that it is set up and you can easily find what you need when you need it.

Now we'll learn how to organize the kitchen by zoning the fridge and pantry to help you more easily prepare and cook meals.

CHAPTER 6

The Organized Kitchen

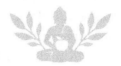

• Kitchen Organization Demystified •

In the previous chapter, we talked about how to zone the kitchen for maximum efficiency. In this chapter, we will talk about overall kitchen organization, then jump into the specifics of organizing the fridge and pantry.

Kitchen organization can truly make or break how you function in the space. If there's too much stuff in the cabinets and you're not putting things away because there's not enough room, then the countertops become cluttered, making it difficult to create a meal because there's insufficient workspace.

That's why we want to act like a restaurant (more about this in Chapter 7) placing anything that's only used for holidays or special occasions in the upper cabinets or in another space altogether. We'll cover more of this throughout the chapter, as well as in Chapter 9: "Get Your Home In Order and Feel Great."

WHAT TOOLS YOU REALLY NEED

An organized kitchen doesn't need all of the gadgets advertisers tell us we need, so it's important to make the distinction between what you THINK you need and what you ACTUALLY need.

Remember, this book is all about simple, healthy eating. That means choosing simple recipes that require fewer pots and pans, plates and utensils—resulting in less cleanup.

To create simple healthy meals, here are the tools you need:

1. A sharp knife. Have at least one sharp knife on hand. Knife blocks that sit on the counter may be nice, but they're naughty when it comes to taking up valuable real estate on your countertops, especially if you have a small kitchen.
2. Cutting board. There are exceptions (if you keep kosher or you're a vegetarian who lives with meat eaters), but typically you only need one sizable cutting board to chop vegetables.
3. Sauté pan. One stainless steel pan is enough to sauté healthy foods. Avoid Teflon-covered pans that can break down after a period of time, releasing toxins in the food you're cooking.
4. Saucepan. You just need one with a lid.
5. Cookie sheet. These are good for roasting vegetables or meats.
6. Mixing bowls. One set of 3 sizes works for baking and cooking.
7. Measuring cups. You just need one set.
8. Measuring spoons. A simple aluminum set works well. Avoid fancy plastic ones and opt for durable tools and can withstand the test of time.
9. Wooden spoon. Good for sautéing veggies in a stainless pan.
10. Spatula. Great for scooping up roasted veggies or flipping meats or tofu in a pan.
11. Tongs. Good for serving spinach or pasta.
12. Slotted spoons. Good for scooping steamed veggies.

Bonus: a kitchen scale that can help when it comes to incorporating portion control as part of a healthy regimen.

• Fresh Fridge •

The fridge is a temporary storage container for foods that need to stay cool.

Over the years, we've seen amazing advancements in refrigerators: Freezers were at the top, then on the left, then at the bottom. Fridges had one door, then two—changes presumably made to create easier access and organization, right?

The good news is you don't need the latest and greatest technology. I'm going to share with you a concept about the refrigerator's purpose that may change the way you think about what you keep in this appliance: the refrigerator is a temporary storage container for food products that require cold temperatures to stay fresh until eaten.

Yup, the fridge is a temporary container. Not a "storage" container. It was introduced as a home appliance in 1913 and was designed to prolong the life of food by keeping it cold. Prior to that, if items needed chilling, they were put in an icebox.

Times were different in the early 1900s. People typically lived within walking distance to the butcher, baker, and candlestick maker. Therefore, foods such as milk, butter, and cheese were purchased (or delivered) and eaten daily, before they expired.

However, the introduction of consumer refrigeration allowed for consistent temperatures, unlike iceboxes, which relied on cooling from blocks of ice that eventually melted and needed replenishing. The consistent temperatures also allowed people to store leftovers confidently, without fear of spoilage, which created more flexibility for families. For example, a family could prepare a large meal and then save time during the week by eating the leftovers. Or they could batch cook and preserve time that way.

This technology changed how people managed their routines, as well as the amount of storage they needed. Instead of a daily trip to the market, they could stock up by only visiting the market a couple times each week.

During this same period of history, people were presented with other new technologies, such as cars, which then allowed them to expand their horizons—literally—by going beyond the neighborhoods they lived in. This meant they could add more items to their grocery carts because they could drive it home instead of carrying or carting it home.

The next major introduction was the idea of suburban living. With all the advancements in technology, families began moving out of cities so they could have more space, which included more storage space. So what do you do when you have space? Fill it!

During this period, people also began acquiring more goods. We'll talk more about this in Chapter 9, "Get Your Home In Order and Feel Great."

My point for taking you back to a time when people were using what they had versus stocking up and needing the space to do it is to show you just how we tend to get ourselves into trouble by "needing" a bigger house, which oftentimes reflects our level of debt and subsequent levels of stress.

How many people do you know who have a stocked fridge and pantry and still go out to dinner five nights a week? It's likely because they are so overwhelmed with the overabundance of choices that they're unable to see through the clutter to make sense of it.

So it's important to return to the idea that the refrigerator is a temporary container for food products that require cold temperatures to stay fresh until eaten. It's NOT a place for food to go to live out its expiration date.

That's why it's essential to have a plan to use the items in the fridge, regularly checking expiration dates along with cleaning and organizing the space, which includes removing everything (shelves too!), wiping it down and returning food items to their designated zones. Doing so helps us make sense of what's available.

We also want to avoid overfilling the fridge, which can create confusion and a "storage" situation versus an in-and-out-flowing of items.

As with anything, you can't fully assess something unless you know exactly what you're working with. Therefore, you need to know what's in every corner of your fridge, and you will by the time we're done with this section.

• Eating Healthier •

To create healthy meals in our kitchen, we must have healthy ingredients on hand. Over the years, I've seen some problems in people's refrigerators, including:

- Produce left in the plastic to rot.
- Not categorizing items.
- Too many boxed or processed food products.
- Unhealthy options, such as sugary desserts.
- Poor organization, including misaligned shelving and putting things in the wrong containers.

All of this generally leads to no healthy cooking in the heart of the home. As mentioned, having too much stuff can create confusion, especially when it's largely unhealthy options. Simple strategies include buying and eating more veggies and reducing or eliminating processed boxed foods.

The process of assessing (inventorying) what you currently have on hand can be challenging and frustrating. But it doesn't have to be. In fact, unless you have the time and budget, I recommend slowly upgrading a couple of items at a time.

Ann's Story

Ann knew her pantry and fridge needed upgrading, but she didn't know where to begin. Her typical routine for shopping did not include a list or a meal plan. And she often went to the supermarket when she was hungry, so making healthier choices wasn't top of mind. Instead, she would grab what she thought she needed. There was no consideration for specific meals and, if there was, it was typically a frozen lasagna dinner or mac-n-cheese. The cart was also typically filled with bags of chips, assorted boxed snacks, case of water and diet soda. The family had a busy schedule, which only made matters worse because they would come home after a long day asking, "What's for dinner?" while peering into a fridge full of unrelated and confusing options, then typically shrug their shoulders while placing an online order for pizza. This repeated routine became stale and they wanted to spice things up by learning the process of meal planning and cooking. First, we cleaned out and organized the fridge and pantry, replacing many of the ingredients that were inflammation-creating. We then followed the meal planning and grocery shopping process to help the family create healthier meals at least five nights a week, which we based on their family goals.

• Inside the Pantry •

Organizing the fridge and pantry means one thing, and filling it with healthier ingredients means another. Combining the two is possible, and I will show you how.

Let's talk about the history of the pantry for a moment. Historically, the pantry was a small utility room in large homes that was primarily used to store serving items, rather than food. Today, however, in less formal environments, the pantry serves as a container (a.k.a. small closet or storeroom) to house non-perishable foods and canned products. It's typically located in the kitchen, but sometimes outside of that space, depending upon the home design. Like the fridge, it's also a temporary container, meant to store items for a period of time, but not permanently. Now if you have space in the pantry for storage of small, countertop appliances or linens you use fairly frequently, designate a shelf or a specific zone for those more permanent items.

Both the pantry and fridge need to rotate the perishable items they house. You can use the FIFO—First In, First Out—method borrowed from accounting terminology, to remember. In this case, it means that whatever items you put in first should be used first. Therefore, when organizing the pantry, create a way to keep the oldest items up front to make sure you use them before replenishing items you may have purchased more recently.

• Getting Started •

Eliminating the unnecessary is essential to avoid confusion and save time. Some call it editing, others call it purging. (We'll learn more about this later.) Use these steps to eliminate unhealthy items from the fridge and pantry:

1. Get rid of packaged items that contain more than five unrecognizable ingredients.
2. Toss expired products and condiments (add the tossed items to a list if you plan to replace them).
3. If you plan to use up what you have instead of tossing or donating, plan to "upgrade" items two at a time when you go to the store.

Pretty simple, right?

• Creating Order and Space for Healthier Foods •

Anytime we want to make progress, it's important to streamline and simplify processes of managing everyday tasks. In this chapter, you will learn how to create order in the fridge and pantry, as well as space for healthier foods.

• Focus on the Fridge •

Amy's Story

Amy's home was beautiful on the surface. But if you opened a closet, pantry, or fridge, it was like entering a different universe. In the fridge, produce regularly rotted in plastic bags and condiments expired. Although Amy went shopping every week, it was a task she just wanted to check off her list. Once she came home from the store and quickly put everything away, without much thought as to where to place it, she was done. She left fruit and vegetables in the plastic produce bags, which meant they typically went to the crisper drawers to die. There was no organization inside the fridge and the quality of food she purchased didn't meet the health and wellness goals she decided she wanted to meet. She hired me to help her organize, save money and to learn how to cook healthy meals. During our initial meeting, we quickly discovered that she had no system for planning. Once we created a meal plan and sorted out her fridge by using the exercises you're about to learn, she was not only able to quickly check grocery shopping off her list, but she was also following the system, which saved her time and fed her family healthy meals each week. This made everyone happier, and mealtime became a truly memorable and pleasant experience filled with conversation and laughter.

• Exercise 1: Zone the Fridge •

To maximize any space, it's important to figure out how you will use, or zone it, asking yourself where will items be placed to make best use of the space? When zoning the fridge, before you remove everything from it, take out a sheet of paper and a pen, pencil, markers, Sharpies, whatever works for you.

Begin by drawing a schematic of the space as if you're looking into the fridge.

Here are the recommended fridge zones:

1. Dairy
2. Fruits and veggies
3. Leftovers
4. Condiments
5. Drinks

HOW ZONING HELPS

Zoning creates spaces for particular categories of items. Therefore, creating zones within your fridge accomplishes several things:

1. You know exactly where to find things AND your family members do, too. Introduce your family members to a system of putting items back where they found them OR if they are the last to use something, to add it to the grocery list.
2. You know when you're running low. This will help you avoid the "I thought we had more of this . . . "
3. Creating a meal from leftovers is simple and easy. If you have a zone for leftovers, you can quickly add those to your weekly Meal Plan.
4. Nothing gets lost at the back of the fridge (and no more unrecognizable smells!)

5. *Mind clutter equals fridge clutter, so organize your Brussel sprouts.*

• Exercise 2: Creating an Organized Fridge •

When we talk about organizing the fridge, it's like organizing any other space, so let's use the GOPACK (Group Objects, Purge, Assign, Contain, and Keep it Up) Method to easily move through the process.

Here's how it works:

Group objects. Put like items together. Let's use condiments as an example. Remove all of them from the fridge and place them on the countertop. Then put all the mustards together, all the pickles in a grouping, etc. Now move to the next step, Purge.

Purge. Once your items are grouped together, this makes it easier to understand what stays and what goes. Using the list above, purge any expired items, items that contain more than five ingredients (all should be recognizable), and toss anything you're planning to put on your upgrade list. Bonus: recycle glass jars by emptying the remaining contents in the trash or garbage disposal, soak the container in hot soapy water, then put in a recycle bin.

Assign. Now it's time to determine where these items will live in your fridge. This is when you pull out the zoning exercise you did earlier and use it to place the items in the chosen locations.

Contain. Once the items are in their assigned spots, you'll now determine what containers, if any, you'll put items in. We do this after we assign so that we don't buy containers we don't need. We also want to make sure the containers we do buy will fit in the drawer or space it will go (make sure to measure).

Tip: Use containers you can label by day of the week. That way, when you come home from shopping, you can immediately put the ingredients that are on your Meal Plan for a particular day directly into the labeled containers.

Keep it up. For maximum efficiency, this process requires maintaining it. Make sure to revisit the GOPAC portion of the GOPACK Method from time to time to keep the highest quality foods in one of the most important—if not the most important—appliance in your home.

CLEAN OUT THE FRIDGE

There's nothing like bringing fresh groceries home and trying to jam them into a disorganized refrigerator full of leftovers and rotting fruits and vegetables. One of the keys to a organized a fridge is to clean it out BEFORE going grocery shopping. This may seem like a hassle, especially if you're pressed for time, so maybe do this the night before. That way you will know exactly what you need and you'll get rid of items that are no longer fresh.

Take these steps to clean out your fridge:

1. Purge. Before your next food shopping trip, prop open the fridge with the trash can. Go through and toss anything outdated, no longer fresh, and any leftovers you know you won't eat (rule of thumb is leftovers should be tossed within three to four days if not eaten). Go ahead, toss them. You won't be struck down by lighting for wasting food. You'll have a chance to redeem yourself in the next few steps.

2. Clean. Pull a few paper towels from the roll and wet them. Wipe out the fridge. You don't need to make this a big production. Just grab, wipe, toss the towels. (You can always do a more thorough cleaning later, but for now, just do it!)

3. Organize. Use the door shelves for jars and condiments. Use the top shelf for things you access regularly if you have a freezer on top. For French door-style refrigerators, use the shelf straight ahead for items you need to access quickly. Designate one shelf for leftovers and put the freshest at the back. Remove your fresh veggies from the bags and organize in containers or the crisper drawers. Put like with like and always put items in the same place.

Not only does this save time, but you'll always know where everything is.

4. Store in glass containers. If you're like me, to save time, you make double and triple batches of food such as rice, steamed or roasted veggies, or black beans. Store them in containers so you can quickly put together a healthy salad. Designate one area of the fridge for these foods for easy access.

• The Purposeful Pantry •

Pat and Cameron's Story

When Pat and Cameron bought their first home, they were still in acquisition mode. The home had three bedrooms, a two-car garage, a large kitchen with walk-in pantry, and more space than they ever had lived in. They were both established in their careers and had a sizable disposable income. They began rapidly filling the home with furniture and accessories. They didn't necessarily consider kitchen organization because they ate dinner out most nights, only using the fridge for leftovers. However, the pantry began to fill up, too, but not with what's traditionally housed in a pantry. Pat and Cameron shopped at a big box store for household items, and since they didn't have much interior storage (and didn't consider the garage for overflow), it went in the pantry. When they had company, the pantry also became the catch-all for items that typically wound up on the kitchen counter, such as mail and craft items purchased and not put away.

The couple decided it was time to cook at home to save money and eat healthier, and they realized they would also need to organize the kitchen in order for it to function well. Most of the kitchen was easy to address because they hadn't overbought on dishes and cookware, but the pantry needed an overhaul. They took my suggestion to put the overflow of toilet paper and paper towels in the garage on easy-to-assemble shelving, create a system for organizing paperwork and mail so it wouldn't accumulate in the kitchen, and began filling the pantry with food-related items.

The pantry is similar to the fridge in that you want it to be a container where items flow in and out regularly. Here are the steps to zone and organize it:

• Exercise 3: Zone the Pantry •

Just like you did with the fridge, zone the pantry by creating a schematic as if you were looking directly it. Now, if there's more than one side or view, draw each separately, but consider them all together. If your pantry is cabinet space, then draw a schematic looking into the space. If it's a deep cabinet with drawers, you may want to consider drawing a schematic as if you're looking down on an open drawer in order to maximize the space available.

Here are the seven recommended zones for the pantry and what you need to know about each one:

Canned Items

What it includes: Anything in a can, of course. Within this category, organize like-items together so you can easily spot when you're running low and add it to your shopping list.
Tip: Use Lazy Susans or stackable shelving to create an organized space.

Baking Items

What it includes: Flour, almond meal, sugar (organic!), brown sugar, other dry goods and used for baking.
Tip: Maintain the freshness of your baking supplies and avoid pesky critters by placing flour, sugar, and so on in sealed, labeled containers.

Pastas/Grains/Cereals

What it includes: Pastas, grains (rice, quinoa, lentils) and cereals.
Tip: Use labeled baskets to separate pastas and grains. Use air-tight containers for cereals.

Condiments

What it includes: Unopened condiments such as mustards, ketchup, red peppers, salsa, etc.
Tip: Organize in a way that you can easily see what you have. Mirror the same organization in the refrigerator for the already-opened condiments; that way you always have a back-up, and when you move one from the pantry to the fridge, you add it to your shopping list.

Beverages

What it includes: Teas, coffees, and bottled or canned overflow
Tip: Remove all from the packaging. Put tea bags in a container (airtight if not separately packaged) and coffee in an airtight container, if not already in one.

Supplies

What it includes: Napkins, paper towels, serving trays, baskets, and cookbooks
Tip: Depending upon the size of the pantry, you may also have room for a recycling bin, cookbooks, and countertop appliances not in use.

Once the pantry is zoned, it's easier to see what you're running low on and when to replenish.

TIPS FOR ZONING THE PANTRY

1. Put more frequently used items at eye level so there's minimal reaching; put supplies on an upper shelf.

2. Avoid zoning a space for things that sit on the floor. Keeping the floor clear allows for easy cleaning. If you do need the space, plan to contain anything that needs to live in that space.
3. Only use the pantry space for kitchen-related items and remember, like with like. Anything related to another home function should go in a storage closet or cabinet in or near where you'll need it.

• Exercise 4: Create an Organized Pantry •

Just as you did for the fridge, use the GOPACK Method to easily move through the process of organizing the pantry:

Group Objects. This is where we put like items together. Let's use baking goods as an example. Remove all the baking goods from the pantry and place them on the countertop, putting all the like items together, such as sugar, flour, brown sugar. Chances are if they weren't organized to begin with, you may have duplicates, so be sure to pull ALL the baking category items out at once. Now move to the next step.

Purge. Once your baking items are grouped together, you can more easily understand what stays and what goes. Using the decision list, purge any expired items, items that contain more than five ingredients (and all should be recognizable), and toss anything you're planning to put on your upgrade list.

Assign. Now it's time to determine where these items will live in your pantry. This is where you pull out the zoning exercise you did earlier and use it to place the items in the chosen locations.

Make it a goal to have all pantry food in clear, air-tight containers—no boxes or manufacturer packaging!

Contain. Once the items are in their assigned spots, determine what you'll put items in, if anything.

There are two reasons contain comes after assign: (1) We need to make sure we don't buy containers for items that don't need containing (Purge) and (2) We want to be sure we buy the correct size containers (Assign).

Use sealed containers for baking items for easy storage and to prevent spillage. This will also help when it comes to identifying what you need to restock. For items such as pastas, use baskets; for canned goods, use Lazy Susans.

Keep it up. For maximum efficiency, this process requires maintenance. Therefore, you'll want to revisit the GOPAC portion of the GOPACK Method from time-to-time to be sure you're keeping the highest quality foods in this space.

TIPS FOR ORGANIZING THE PANTRY

1. Group like items together on pantry shelves.
2. Use the GOPAC part of the method before buying containers.
3. Put baking items in airtight containers to maximize space and prevent items from going bad.
4. Use eye level space for most frequently used items.
5. Store seldom-used counter appliances on upper shelves.
6. Keep uncontained items off the floor. If you need to use the floor space for any storage, contain the items so you can easily remove them to clean the floor space.

TIPS FOR STOCKING THE PANTRY

- Leave room for growth—don't jam-pack it full.
- Remember the 80/20 rule that states we only use twenty percent of what we own. We're simply providing storage

for the rest. Imagine what life would be like with eighty percent less of what we manage on a daily basis? (See the High Cost of Clutter exercise in Chapter 9).

- Store extra supplies, such as paper towels and napkins, on upper shelves.
- Be deliberate about the use of the space.
- Put things away in the proper places.

CONTAINING YOUR PANTRY ITEMS

To fully organize your pantry, it's always nice to use containers as a finishing touch. In the pantry, specifically, use air-tight containers that are clear AND LABELED, so you can easily spot what you need.

As mentioned earlier, Mason jars are also useful. They're easy to find at big box stores, the grocery store, or online. Some people find the tops a nuisance because there are two pieces, but I like them because they are extremely affordable, you can typically buy them at your grocery store, and they are easy to label. You can get Mason jars with a single lid too.

Containers are great for bulk items, so if you purchase things like rolled oats, quinoa, or rice in bulk, you can purchase exactly how much will fit into your jars. Some people even take the jars with them when they go to the store. I do encourage you to use what's in the pantry, then replenish. If you go to the store weekly, then there's typically no need to over-buy and over-stock.

• Practice Upgrading: Healthier Substitutes •

Allison's Story

After having a few setbacks with some of her favorite junk food items, Allison quickly realized that if she kept it in the house, she would eat it! This motivated her to research healthier options that she could snack on without sacrificing the hard work she was putting in by reducing sugar and eliminating processed foods.

To her surprise, Allison found many healthy upgrades that allowed her to enjoy a splurge without the chemicals and calories. For example, she loves ice cream, but realized dairy wasn't helping her efforts to improve digestion. She found a non-dairy ice cream that satisfied her craving and left her content instead of bloated and later experiencing a sugar crash.

As far as the condiments in the fridge, there are lots of healthy substitutes. Instead of the syrup you get in a plastic bottle along with chemicals and too much bad sugar (high-fructose corn syrup), try pure maple syrup. And remember, you don't need that much syrup when it's pure. Instead of putting the bottle on the table when you have pancakes, give everyone a shot glass with a tablespoon of syrup. It'll be their own personal sized portion!

The word "upgrade" signifies something better than what you already have. For example, getting upgraded to first class when we check in for a flight. Or, an upgrade may be that when you receive a salary increase or a bonus, you discontinue using one makeup brand and upgrade to something that costs more, but does a better job with skin management. Or you could upgrade a membership from basic to premium. You get the gist. And this is what we want to do when it comes to our health and what we're eating—upgrade!

Here is a list of upgrades that you can incorporate now to start eating healthier—and start loving the body you live in.

These are the most commonly used items and the healthier versions you can upgrade to.

Current Product	Healthier Version
Vegetable Oil	Olive Oil, Avocado Oil
Spices	Fresh or Organic Spices
Butter	Coconut Oil or Earth Balance
Margarine	Grass-fed Butter
Sour Cream	Greek Yogurt
Pancake Syrup	Pure Maple Syrup
Sugar	Raw Sugar, Organic Sugar, Stevia, Agave
Ice Cream	Organic Coconut Bliss or Home-made Banana Ice Cream
Milk Chocolate	Organic Dark Chocolate
Meat	Organic, Antibiotic-free Meat
Velveeta or Packaged Cheese	Organic Cheese, Cashew Cheese
Creamer or Half-n-Half	So Delicious Coconut Milk
Milk	Almond Milk, Coconut Milk

• Exercise 5: Creating the Ultimate Healthy Kitchen •

We all want a kitchen that is truly functional—easy to get in and out of—and one that we enjoy. There are some simple steps you can take to feel more organized in your space. Making these changes, whether you spend ten minutes or ten hours, will help. So this is more of a challenge than an exercise, but one you should be able to accomplish quite easily.

Plan to spend at least one hour on this exercise. You may need more or less time, depending upon the current state of your kitchen, which is perfectly okay. When you organize a space, always leave room to grow (as a rule of thumb, twenty to twenty-five percent).

Creating the ultimate healthy kitchen involves incorporating at least three of the following suggestions into your kitchen. Go through the list first, then choose three.

1. Place items where you use them. This should be relatively simple if you've completed the zoning exercise. For instance, put the pots and pans in the lower cabinets closest to the stove, and place the spices in the upper cabinets directly next to the stove or nearby.

2. Eliminate duplicates. If you have more than one set of everyday dishes, consider rotating them with the seasons to unclutter your cabinet space. Store extras or, better yet, donate or give them away.

3. Incorporate Lazy Susans to increase cabinet space. This spinner works great for spices or canned goods. Pull-down spice racks also work well—they keep spices in place and allow you to take advantage of vertical shelf space.

4. Toss or replace chipped glassware. Now, this doesn't mean going down the rabbit hole of shopping for new glassware.

This means staying focused on this challenge, assessing what you have, then planning out some time to research or shop for new glassware. For a family of four, have at least eight to ten glasses, perhaps different sizes, but no need to go overboard because if you implement a system of washing up every night and/or running the dishwasher, then you'll have enough for each day.

5. Clean out the refrigerator and freezer on a regular basis. Performing this task prior to going food shopping is a great way to make space for the fresh items you'll bring home. Use the zones we established earlier to effectively organize the space.

6. Organize with guests in mind. If someone was staying in your home and you weren't there, could they easily find what they needed? Does your kitchen organization make sense so if someone was looking for a drinking glass, they could easily find one?

7. Countertops are not for storage. Clear the decks! Countertops are valuable real estate in your kitchen. They are meant as a workspace to prepare food and keep appliances that are used regularly (for example, a coffee pot or toaster). If you're using countertops to house items that are not used regularly, you want to consider purging items in the cabinets to make room for relocating non-kitchen items to another part of the house. For example, put paperwork in the office or projects in closed storage in the playroom.

Circle three from the list above and go for it! If you're an overachiever (wink, wink) and have a lot of time, then choose more, or break it up over a couple of days.

• Mindless vs. Mindful •

Mindless: Buying vegetables, leaving them in plastic bags, then putting the bags directly in the refrigerator.

Mindful: Going to the grocery store or farmers market with reusable vegetable bags, returning home, removing them from the bag and placing them in the vegetable zone in the fridge.

Now it's time to learn how to simplify the process of planning, prepping, and serving simple, healthy meals.

CHAPTER 7

Meal Planning and Preparation

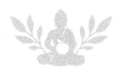

IN THIS CHAPTER, WE'LL cover Meal Planning 101, Meal Planning Tools, Grocery Shopping Strategies, and Meal Preparation. We uncover the four elements to simplify grocery shopping and learn how to reduce your grocery budget and prepare food and cook in batches. We'll also go over what to buy in bulk and how to decide when to buy online or at farmer's markets and co-ops.

Meal planning is the deciding what you'll eat and creating a schedule. Meal preparation is prepping and cooking the food. Creating healthier meals isn't as challenging or time-consuming as you might think, especially if you've followed the guidance in the previous chapters, which has helped you gain knowledge and confidence. Now that you've learned the basics of nutrition and you've organized your kitchen, it's time to learn how to effectively plan meals, optimize your grocery shopping efforts, and prepare meals to improve the quality of food you're eating and minimize the time spent preparing it during the week.

You've also created systems. And remember, SYSTEM stands for Saving You Serious Time, Energy, and Money. Over time, systems become more effective because you tweak and fine tune, making them more efficient. Therefore, once a kitchen is properly zoned, organized, and stocked with healthier food choices, the process becomes easier to manage and improve over time.

Now you're way ahead of the game and ready to take your health to the next level. Learning how to meal plan and shop so you can eat meals will give you more energy and save you time and money that could be spent on other areas of your life you want focus on improving. Also, by incorporating healthy upgrades, you'll be on your way to a healthier lifestyle in no time!

• Preparation •

The key to any successful event is the preparation.

Without proper preparation, we spend more money, buy the wrong products, forget ingredients, and, if I may I say it again, spend more money than necessary.

When it comes to planning, an analogy I like to use is wedding planning because of all the details involved. Unless you have an unlimited budget (and sometimes not even then) everything doesn't magically fall into place after you've said "yes" and booked a venue. There are checklists and menus, bar considerations, desserts, floral arrangements, decorations, signage, and more. Sometimes there's a wedding planner, but in our context of meal planning, the wedding planner may be replaced with a health and wellness coach or nutritionist.

In other words, there's work to do for any worthwhile "event," but I'm going to super-simplify the process for you so it feels more like a task than an event—and a successful one at that!

• Using Time Wisely Is Everything •

Well-planned events require paying attention to timing. In the case of eating healthier, this includes when you decide to grocery shop or, based on your busy schedule, shopping online after the kids have gone to sleep and picking up the order the following day.

Also, taking time each week to meal plan can make shopping easier because you're considering breakfast, lunch, dinner, and snacks—you can easily shop once, prepare things in advance, and pack a healthy lunch if you work outside the home or you're running errands.

This will help you keep it clean when it comes to your daily choices. Moving forward in this chapter, we will discuss in detail how to plan meals, including snacks, and how to create a solid shopping list and effectively grocery shop.

To begin, you'll need to determine:

- The budget.
- How many people you will feed.
- How many days you're buying for.
- What meals you'll cook (use recipe books or online sources).

Before we dive into the nuts and bolts of how to plan meals and grocery shop, there are several other topics I want to cover that can help you not only make better choices, but understand why.

• Act Like a Restaurant •

If you've worked in food service, especially in a kitchen, you'll understand this more quickly. Although I haven't worked in a restaurant, I have a number of family members who have, and I also appreciate efficiency and simplicity, so I've paid attention to how well-run kitchens operate.

Imagine entering a restaurant and ordering a veggie sandwich with a bowl of chicken noodle soup and they have nothing prepared. The cook would need to start from scratch, beginning with boiling water, preparing and cooking chicken, cutting vegetables, taking toppings for the sandwich out of the fridge, cooking the noodles, simmering the chicken noodle soup, etc. You get the picture! It would take a long time to get your food delivered to your table or put into a to-go bag.

Too long to be truly efficient and serve all the customers that come in and out every day.

If we think how most restaurants operate, they do food prep, so when someone places an order, the kitchen staff are taking the ingredients they've already prepared and assembling them into the sandwich they are making or the soup they are serving.

To create simple, healthy meals at home, we want to be equally efficient, having key ingredients prepared so putting together a healthy meal doesn't take very long. Therefore, keep in mind the efficiency of a kitchen restaurant. Use a specific day/time for food preparation so that during the week, you are doing a little cooking but mainly assembling a healthy meal.

Here's an example. If you roast a chicken on Sunday, you could use some for a salad topping on Monday and a main protein on Tuesday. Or if you make roasted vegetables, those could be a topping for a Buddha bowl, where all you need to do when you arrive home after work is toss some rice or quinoa into a rice cooker (or maybe you already have that prepared too), then assemble your healthy dish.

As with any system, you can and should tweak them over time, making it more efficient and, in this case, healthier.

• Choosing the Right Recipes •

We're all different, so even the recipes I've included at the back of the book may not resonate with you. That's okay. It's up to you to discover what you love. You can begin with the Determine Your Taste exercise at the end of this chapter to help you understand what to keep in your pantry and fridge. Google has also made it incredibly easy to find recipes that contain what you like, so look there too. But don't get caught up on recipes that are complicated and require hours to make. Leave those for a rainy weekend when you can experiment in more detail.

It's important to remember that we're all responsible for our own health and it will be necessary for you to do some of the heavy lifting to determine what you like and how to make it.

Start by incorporating only a few new healthy recipes each month. If you do only three simple recipes each month, at the end of the year, you'll have thirty-six recipes, which would give you plenty of variety every month after that. You could even create a family cookbook at the end of the year to celebrate your healthier living quest.

Instead of choosing complicated recipes, add items to your pantry and fridge that you like to eat. For example, if you have a sweet tooth and love chocolate, try a healthy chocolate option such as Raw Chocolate Balls, which are made with four simple ingredients: almond meal, cacao powder, vanilla, and pure maple syrup. Stock your pantry with these items for a quick recipe that satisfies a craving for chocolate and your sweet tooth.

• What If It Doesn't Come Out Right? •

Anytime we learn something new or make a change in how we do something, there's a learning curve. This curve presents us with challenges and setbacks, which is totally normal. Learning involves failure—it's a natural part of the process. One of the best examples I heard not too long ago is that when a baby is learning to walk, they fall down and get back up—they don't stop trying until they've mastered walking. Give yourself a pat on the back for trying something new, keep a sense of humor, and go with it. Eventually you'll get it.

• Why Healthy Food Doesn't Taste Good •

I can't tell you the number of times I've heard people say, "I'd like to eat healthier, but healthy food doesn't taste good!" I find this humorous on one hand because oftentimes an adult can sound like a five-year-old who doesn't want to try something new or who is convinced that what they are being offered will taste bad.

The real reason healthier foods sometimes don't taste very good is that when we've been eating a "diet" of largely processed foods, our taste buds have become accustomed to the taste of what are actually chemical ingredients—not real food.

As mentioned in Nutrition 101, in order for boxed foods to maintain a long-lasting shelf life, it's necessary for food "manufacturers" (that is a clue right there!) to add preservatives to the food. These tend to be forms of sugar and sodium, along with other types of chemicals. Although we think something tastes good, it's only because that's what we are used to. Therefore, it's important to give your taste buds an opportunity to acclimate to healthier, nutrient-rich foods.

Moving toward healthier eating takes some steps. The first step is understanding more clearly what you like to eat. If it's burgers and fries, then start by upgrading the ingredients you use. Make homemade burgers with organic meat. Perhaps bake them instead of frying them. Or if you're a pasta eater, instead of choosing the spaghetti you've been grabbing randomly, try a quinoa pasta instead and a lower-sodium red pasta sauce.In Exercise 1 at the end of this chapter, you can explore what tastes good to you and identify the patterns and indulgences.

• Meal Planning 101 •

Keeping in mind the learning curve, the initial transition to meal planning may feel awkward and even frustrating. If you're able to grasp the idea that taking the time to plan for the week will then free up time to focus on other things, that may help you through the initial learning. Again, like anything else, until you've worked through a process several times, it will feel foreign, awkward, and not so much fun. The flipside, however, is that when you consistently work this meal planning muscle you will be strong and have a tool that will serve you and your family very well.

Another important thing to remember here is that getting into the kitchen is key to eating healthier. Our society has become accustomed to fast food, ordering in, and essentially not preparing our own food. And this is problematic because unless you cook for yourself, you really don't know what's in the food. The only way to be sure you're in control of your healthy eating journey is to do more healthy food prep and cooking.

The simplified method of meal planning I'm about to introduce is all about creating simple, healthier meals. Start slow and gradually work toward improving your skills.

• Getting Started: Meal Planning Tools •

Getting started can be the hardest part. Procrastination and indecision are the killjoys that lead to never getting anything done. So, best to take on the attitude that done is better than perfect! Put aside your trepidation about doing it perfectly, throw caution to the wind, and get a move on.

You will need the following items:

- Meal planner form (available at the end of this chapter and at www.mindbodykitchenbook.com)
- Family/personal calendar (a written calendar or one on your smartphone)
- Shopping list (use the notes section of your phone or a piece of paper)

• Tips •

Plan for leftovers. Give yourself a night off by making extra, then save the leftovers for either the next night or two nights later.

Lower your expectations. When you're learning something new, it's not always easy and it takes time to adopt new habits and routines. Give yourself a break by keeping your expectations low and keeping it simple, which means avoid complicated recipes. As I mentioned earlier, save those for when you have all day to cook and experiment.

• Grocery Shopping •

Jane's Story

Once Jane became a mom, she worked part-time from home while her kids attended daycare and pre-school. It was at this time that grocery shopping became a challenge. Taking her kids to the store took a lot of effort and she would often spend too much money because mystery items would wind up in the cart. Jane decided that although she would like to choose her own produce and other items, having someone else do that was an easier option than going to the store herself. And if it didn't work out, she could always find another solution. So she started ordering her groceries online. This also helped her plan meals more effectively because she could make sure she had all the ingredients already on hand or, if not, add them to her virtual shopping cart. She would also save money because it was easier to avoid buying impulse items.

Jane would finish up work at home, get in the car, pick up the kids from school, and leisurely drive to the grocery store where an attendant would load the groceries into her car. By that time, her kids would fall asleep for their naps. Sometimes Jane would even zip through the Starbucks drive-through for a coffee.

Jane figured out a way to make everyone happy when it came to food shopping.

When she arrived home with the groceries, the kids typically continued their naps, which gave Jane time to put the groceries away and check email. Once the kids were up, they could enjoy some outdoor play and ease into the evening in a relaxed way.

This created ease in Jane's day and she embraced it!

So, my suggestion is to make a grocery list and do what works best for you and your family. If this means ordering online or taking a trip to the store, then plan it around other related activities so you can maximize your time.

We'll get to your personalized Grocery Store Shopping Strategies soon, but here are some informational points to read before you refine your strategy:

Food manufacturers pay a premium for shelf space. So the manufacturers with the most dollars will have products on end-caps and at eye level. Also keep in mind they put the foods they're trying to sell to children at their eye level, so you may want to rethink whether you take the little ones with you or keep them in the cart while shopping.

Shop the perimeter. By shopping the perimeter and avoiding the interior of the food store, by default you make healthier choices. Typically you'll find the freshest food on the outskirts of the store.

Spend most of your time in the produce section. By incorporating more produce into your daily diet, you will by default become healthier and likely drop a few pounds, if that's your thing.

Use reusable bags. Eliminating plastic and reusing bags will help reduce waste. Contribute to the good of Mother Earth, please.

Don't purchase bottled water. Yes, we want to drink more water, but in reusable cups. These one-time disposable water "bottles" have proven to cause more harm than good, with ocean pollution on the rise.

Buy organic whenever possible. By default, if you do this, you will be healthier, especially with meat products. Remember, you're ingesting whatever the animal ate while they were being raised.

Use the Clean Fifteen/Dirty Dozen. This is a suggested list of the fruits and vegetables you should buy organic or not. Again, by default, if you follow this list, you will be eating healthier.

Use fresh ingredients, avoiding processed packets of mixtures. I used to be a big fan of a packaged product that would allow me to make an alfredo dish. Now I make dishes like Avocado Fettuccine with fresh ingredients that include whole-grain pasta, avocado, onions, garlic, pepper, salt, and a variety of spices. Create a healthier version of a dish you love.

• Benefits of Online Shopping •

As I mentioned in Jane's story, online shopping allowed her to create ease in her day. There are many other advantages to online shopping too:

- Eliminate impulse buying. There's a better chance you'll stick to the list while filling your online cart.

- Help with meal planning. We've all gone to the store and forgotten an ingredient due to distractions or not have a complete list. Or we're missing something at home so we need to make a last-minute trip to complete a recipe.

- Save time traveling to the store. If you're picking up groceries in your car, this may not save you time, but if you have them delivered or order online, that's a time saver!

- Convenience. You can shop anytime during the day.

- Saved shopping lists. If you develop a certain repertoire or like to prepare similar meals over and over again, this is especially handy!

- Use several sources. Shopping local and national sources can help if you are in an area with limited access to healthier ingredients. For example, Thrive.com and Vitacost.com sell ingredients you may not find in mainstream grocery stores.

• Meal Preparation •

As I mentioned at the beginning of this chapter, when we're prepared, things more likely go off without a hitch, we have time in our schedule to breathe, and we have the option to incorporate other positive and mindful ways to step up our health game. Meal prep allows us to quickly prepare dinner on a Tuesday because we've prepped food on Sunday, which would then allow us to incorporate a spontaneous family bike ride after dinner or a walk in the evening without having spent an hour and a half preparing, cooking, and cleaning up. Meal prep provides a double bonus of healthy eating and more time to do what you want.

When you begin meal prep, you'll have already completed your meal planning and grocery shopping, which you will want to do either the day of or the day before.

Choose a day/time during the week that allows for at least two hours. For many, this would be a Sunday afternoon, but it certainly doesn't have to be that for everyone. So choose your "Sunday."

SET A TIMER

With anything task-related, setting a timer can truly keep you focused on accomplishing what you set out to do. Parkinson's Law states that a task expands to the time available, which means if you give yourself two hours, it will likely take two hours and if you give yourself an hour, you'll likely accomplish what you set out to do in an hour. It's all relative, so be realistic, but set a timer.

If you weren't able to accomplish the task during the set time, you can review, reassess and make tweaks to make adjustments moving forward. Remember, the process of becoming more efficient takes time, so allow yourself the space to create and fine-tune a system.

When I was in college, there was always a debate about studying and listening to music. I found I needed quiet, and others couldn't study if they weren't listening to some background noise. But when I'm cooking, I love to listen to music. It feels fun, and there's always an opportunity for a brief dance party while chopping vegetables (best to put the knife down while shaking your booty, however). You may also want to incorporate some fun while food prepping this to make the time fly by a little more quickly.

Always keep in mind that by continually reassessing a process and system, you can improve and make them more efficient over time. Just give yourself the time and periodically reflect on the improvements you've made.

ELIMINATE DISTRACTIONS

If you are easily distracted, see what you can do to eliminate the distractions, then break down the steps into little chunks. For example, when I make a recipe, I take all the ingredients and line them up in the order that they are added to the recipe. Once I add the ingredients, I move it to another location on the counter to make sure I don't get confused. That way if I do become distracted, I can easily regroup knowing where I left off.

If you have small children, you may want to use nap time for food preparation. If you know your energy level is higher in the morning, then that may be the best time. I don't know you personally, so unless we had a discussion and I visited your kitchen, it's really not possible for me to identify what your distractions are. And, besides, we're empowered when we take notice of our surroundings, view them objectively, identify issues, and then make the necessary shifts to function in a way that's best for us.

If you need support, however, ask a trusted friend to point out what they see as distractions. This would be someone who doesn't live with you so they're not "blind" to your surroundings; after a while, we all become a little used to our surroundings. If you need more assistance than your friend can give, hire a professional organizer. If I'm not able to come to your home due to physical distance, consider a virtual session with me to assess and organize your kitchen for healthier eating.

You can do this!

• Batch Cooking •

Batch cooking involves creating food that is for more than one meal or a combination of meals. You could batch cook on a Sunday, for example, and make enough vegetables for three different meals during the week, or meat for two meals. Batch cooking is done once you've filled out your meal plan form and shopped for the ingredients.

WHAT YOU NEED

In a typical batch cooking scenario, have the following tools on hand:

1. Sharp knife
2. Cutting board
3. Peeler
4. Colander
5. Cookie sheet
6. Parchment paper
7. Pot with lid
8. Food to prepare, which could consist of a bag of carrots, a head of broccoli, half a dozen chicken breasts, lettuce for a salad.
9. Containers for the individually prepared items.

STEP ONE

Peel and prep the vegetables for roasting and/or steaming.

STEP TWO

Roast/bake or steam.

<u>STEP THREE</u>

Separate cooked food into containers to store in the fridge (in the prepared food zone) and eat according to your meal plan for the week.

These steps will save time and also help you easily pack up lunches and assemble meals quickly when you come home from work.

Note: Batch cooking will potentially save you a few hours each week. However, keep in mind that once you cook food, the nutrients begin depleting. Therefore, if you want to get maximum nutrition from your food source, consider chopping on prep-day and cooking the day you plan to eat the food, allowing a little extra time for this process. Do keep in mind though that if you haven't been eating many vegetables, you're still winning if you're cooking the vegetables a few days in advance! So weigh the nutrient/time ratio carefully. Or start by prepping and cooking, then once you have that process down, prep on one day and cook the day of. Remember, small steps equal big results. Master one process, then move to another.

• Exercise 1: Mindful Eating: Taste & Time •

There are absolutely no right or wrong answers here! And please do not apply self-judgment. This exercise is to help you get truly comfortable with the types of foods you enjoy and THEN create healthier versions so you can satisfy cravings—whether sweet or savory (or both)—and enjoy what you eat.

1. What tastes do you like most?

    ❑ Sweet
    ❑ Savory
    ❑ Salty
    ❑ Sour
    ❑ Bitter

2. Describe your taste for the items you checked off. For example,
    if you like sweets, what exactly are your favorite types of
    sweets? Donuts or chocolate ice cream, Sour Patch Kids or
    Twizzlers?

    _____

    _____

    _____

    _____

    _____

3. Do you eat meat? If so, what are your favorite types?
    For example, red meat that's grilled or chicken that's fried?

    _____

    _____

    _____

    _____

    _____

4. Do you enjoy eating vegetables? What types? For example,
    frozen vegetables that are steamed, fresh vegetables that are
    roasted? Veggies mixed in with stew or in a casserole? Or
    none at all?

    _____

    _____

    _____

    _____

    _____

5. Is evening snacking a thing for you? Describe your favorite snacks, when you like to eat them, and how frequently. Also enter the times of day/evening you snack. For example, do you crave chips or ice cream while watching TV at 10 p.m.?

_____

_____

_____

_____

_____

6. Describe your favorite type of breakfast. For example, cereal with milk, glazed donuts, a fried egg?

_____

_____

_____

_____

What do you love about this favorite breakfast? How does it make you feel? For example, are you not a morning person so grabbing a donut or bagel does the trick, or do you watch the news while eating breakfast?

_____

_____

_____

_____

7. Describe your favorite lunch food and where/how you eat it.
    For example, are you so busy at work that you grab something
    quick and eat while you work?

    _____

    _____

    _____

    _____

    _____

What do you love about this favorite lunch? How does it make you
feel? For example, lunch is a time when you get to catch up with
work friends or take a break mid-day.

    _____

    _____

    _____

    _____

    _____

8. Describe your favorite type of dinner. For example, going out
    to eat with family or friends, a warm meal with lots of spices
    and tastes, or a quick microwave meal that simply fills you up.

    _____

    _____

    _____

    _____

What do you love about this favorite dinner? How does it make you feel? Food surrounds a lot of celebrations. Does your favorite meal evoke feelings of celebration or is it purely a function of eating something to make you feel full?

_____

_____

_____

_____

_____

9. Do you notice any patterns or common food choices? For example, do you tend toward savory or sweet foods? Do certain foods or particular meals trigger specific emotions? Are their memories associated with certain meals?

_____

_____

_____

_____

_____

_____

_____

_____

For many, there are lots of emotions surrounding the food choices we make.

What have you learned about yourself from this exercise? How can you take what you've learned and make adjustments to your current habits and routines?

_____

_____

_____

_____

_____

• Exercise 2: Meal Planning 101 •

Now let's make a meal plan. Grab your Meal Planning tools, sit in a comfortable spot, take a deep breath, and follow these instructions below.

Step One: Take out your Meal Planner form.

Step Two: Determine your budget for the week.

If you've never really created a grocery budget, you can do so by simply reviewing your bank statements to see how much money you've been spending at the grocery store. This would include all trips, such as last-minute items you forgot, to your weekly or bi-weekly haul. Calculate how much you spend in a month and divide by four to get a weekly number. Use this number initially as a baseline. You'll likely tweak this as you move forward, which is expected.

Step Three: Look at your calendar and, using the Meal Planner form, immediately cross off the days you will not cook due to out-of-the-home commitments. For example, if you have dinner out scheduled with friends, then cross that off. If you have a breakfast meeting with clients, cross that off. Also, initially, you may want to choose a night off too while you adjust to this new system. But continue to use your newfound knowledge to choose healthier and nutritious foods.

Step Four: Determine how many people will be eating at each meal. Make a notation in each box.

Step Five: Choose simple recipes for the days you will prepare meals. You can use the Three-Day Jumpstart at the back of this book as a simple way to ease into this new lifestyle, then incorporate new meals.

Step Six: Create a shopping list. If you use the Three-Day Jumpstart, that comes with a shopping list. You may need to adjust the quantities based on the number of people you're feeding. The Jumpstart typically feeds two to three people for three to five days.

Now it's time to shop! Whether at home or online, you will be armed with what you need.

Week of: _____

Meal Planner Form

10. Determine your budget $_____
11. Determine the days you'll be meal/snack prepping—Cross off any days/time where food is provided.
12. Determine number of people _____
13. Choose recipes—select simple recipes to begin, using healthier ingredients. Keep it simple! Leave complicated recipes for a planned day when you have a lot of time.
14. Create shopping list

	Sun	Mon	Tues	Wed	Thurs	Fri	Sat
Break-fast							
Snack							
Lunch							
Snack							
Dinner							

• Exercise 3: Your Grocery Shopping Strategies •

This exercise will help you further hone in on your personalized grocery shopping strategies. The overall goal is to save time, energy, and money, and to avoid last-minute trips to the grocery store or worse, through the drive-through!

This exercise is divided into three sections:

1. What you need for the grocery store
2. Where to put your supplies for the grocery store
3. How to efficiently tackle the grocery store

What you need

When you physically go to the grocery store, you'll want to have the following in hand:

- A shopping list (created during meal planning).
- Coupons. For some this can create more work, so weigh the amount of time it takes to accomplish the task of coupon clipping, whether you actually enjoy it, and if it saves you money on healthier items.
- Eco-friendly reusable bags. Once you've brought your haul home, return the bags to your car so you're prepared for next time.
- A full stomach. Shopping on an empty stomach can result in impulse purchases.

Now answer these questions for optimum efficiency.

1. Do you have your shopping lists printed and ready to fill out when you're planning your meals? Be sure to take a list to the store! This is important. If you're following the meal planning steps, which will help you become more efficient, you will absolutely save more time, energy and money. So,

follow the steps and make sure to have your shopping list with you whether you go to a brick and mortar store or shop online.

2. Are you a Coupon Queen or more of a rogue shopper? There's no right or wrong answer. They key is to identify what you're actually willing to do. Some may think they should be a coupon clipper because their mom was or their friends do it. I highly encourage you to determine if this is an activity you enjoy, because if it's not, then you are wasting time on a low-energy task when you could put high-energy toward researching healthier food options.

3. Do you have reusable bags that are foldable, convenient, and that you really enjoy using? Now don't go on a shopping spree to buy reusable bags. This is not a task to distract you, but one to make you more efficient. If you have reusable bags in your possession and you're okay with them, use them! If you prefer the ones that fold up into a nice little case, then go buy them. But again, weigh the time, energy, and money you're expending on this task.

• Mindless vs. Mindful •

Mindless: Stocking up on unhealthy snacks because they are on sale.

Mindful: Researching healthy snack options and stocking up on those instead.

Next we'll learn how a healthy home is just as important as a healthy body. There are plenty of chemicals lurking under the cabinets and in our laundry detergents, so it's important to clean this up too!

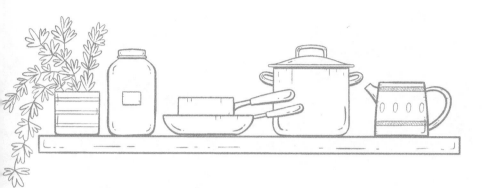

Part Three

CREATING A HEALTHY HOME

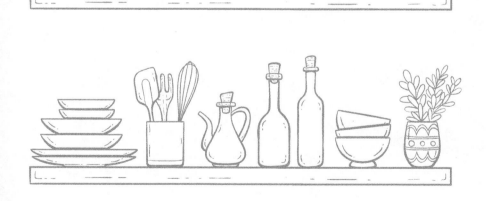

CHAPTER 8

Detoxing Your Home

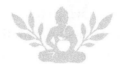

CREATING A HEALTHY HOME starts with detoxing your home. This chapter focuses on identifying and eliminating the toxins that are hiding in your home. In earlier chapters, we discussed how you can essentially detox the body by reducing and eliminating processed foods and incorporating healthier options—the internal. Now, over the next two chapters, we'll cover toxins in the home and the external effects toxins and clutter have on us—the external.

If you're feeling overwhelmed at this point, it's understandable. But you've read this far and you're still here, so that's a great sign. You're becoming aware of how you will create a healthier you, a healthy kitchen, and a healthier home. When clutter accumulates—whatever form it's in—it takes time to undo. Reducing and eliminating starts with awareness. Now that you've got that, you can begin to break down your health journey into manageable goals, using the techniques we've already covered. Let's proceed to the toxins that are hiding in your home and how to eliminate them.

• What Toxins Are Hiding In Your Home? •

Did you know that most households contain more than sixty toxic products? Yep, everything from cleaning supplies and laundry detergents to cosmetics and over-the-counter medications. And that's just what we put near or in and on our bodies. There are also household products like WD-40 and Goo Gone lurking under our cabinets and creating a toxic environment.

While it has become more commonplace to read the ingredients labels on food products, we still aren't paying more attention to reading the ingredients labels on products we put on our skin and in our bodies.

Several years ago, I was having trouble sleeping. I was doing all the right things in terms of a bedtime routine. Winding down with a cup of tea and engaging in some quiet time by reading a book. I had removed the TV from my bedroom long before that and I was avoiding the use of a smartphone to fall asleep, instead using deep breathing techniques. Still, I was having trouble falling asleep and not sleeping well once I did.

One day while washing my sheets and pouring bleach into the washing machine, it occurred to me that maybe it was the bleach. I chucked to myself and said out loud, "You haven't figured this one out before now?!" Bleach is a toxic chemical that's used to disinfect. It's also used to power wash homes, clean up blood in an emergency room, and more. But, for me, like many others, bleach was a familiar scent that was part of my childhood and then my adulthood. My grandmother always washed whites with bleach and so did my mother. It was a scent of cleanliness. That particular day, however, I asked myself, "Is it really wise to wash sheets and towels in bleach?" The answer was a very clear no!

Once I stopped using bleach and switched to a milder, fragrance-free laundry detergent, I immediately began sleeping better and my skin irritations and allergic reactions stopped. My sinuses no longer suffered, either.

Years before that epiphany, I began to develop a sensitivity to other smells and fragrances. Reflecting back on these experiences, I now believe it was my body's way of telling me I needed to "clean up" my product choices and use more natural ones. I also stopped using dryer sheets, as well as cleaning products containing harsh chemicals. The nose knows best!

• Allergy Issues On the Rise •

Allergy testing is alive and well today. In fact, a quick Google search will show that the industry brought in $1.3 billion in 2015 and is expected to triple to $3.8 billion by 2024. People are running to allergists for diagnoses, but they aren't clearing out the chemicals in their food, cosmetics, and cleaning products. Imagine the time and money we could save by becoming more mindful and removing toxic food, cleaning products, and other potential allergens first.

Before you head out the door and get poked and prodded and have things stuck up your nose by an allergist, ask yourself what you can clean up when it comes to what you eat, the cosmetic products you use, and the cleaning products that are hiding in your cabinets. What toxins can you eliminate?

• Eliminating Toxins in the Home •

Our home is our sanctuary. It's not only important, but necessary and vital to our health to live in a toxin-free environment so we can relax and feel our best. We became intensely aware of this in 2020 when the pandemic hit, and we were forced to be home twenty-four hours a day, seven days a week. People began rethinking how they use their spaces, and home organization became important because it was necessary to create dedicated workspaces and schooling spaces for our families. Home renovations increased too after people realized they could utilize the footprint of their homes more effectively and efficiently.

We'll discuss decluttering and organization in Chapter 9, so let's get back to the toxins and how we can eliminate them. Here are some simple strategies to get some instant results:

Under the kitchen sink. Remove harsh chemicals and make a switch to more natural products. Choose one brand of cleaning products. Or if you want to go all-natural, you can replace much of what's under the kitchen sink with vinegar, baking soda, and drops of essential oils to make the home smell good. In fact, tea tree oil acts as a natural disinfectant. Organize products in a cleaning caddy. You'll solve your primary goal of eliminating toxins, and you'll also get you organized so you can efficiently zip through cleaning your spaces.

Under the bathroom sink. Put a basket about the size of a shoebox under your bathroom sink or nearby. After you use a product—either cosmetic or cleaning—put it in the basket. Do this for a week. Then eliminate all other products that live under your sink. You can use this strategy for the draws and shelves too. The goal is to determine what you're actually using on a regular basis and closely scrutinize whether you need all of the other products taking up space. If you're not ready to purge, at least remove what's not being used from the top of the vanity to unclutter that space, which will make wiping down the countertops quick and easy. We already walked through how to decide where to shop for groceries. You can do the same when buying skincare products. Just like with food, higher quality products without chemicals may cost more, but if you're using less—and not constantly "shopping" for the next best thing—you're detoxing your skin *and* saving money. This can also help you to focus on a regimen that has fewer steps and is gentler on your skin.

The medicine cabinet. Responsibly eliminate all expired medications and medications you're no longer taking. If you were prescribed a medication for an ailment that no longer exists, toss it. Separate prescriptions from other over-the-counter items to avoid any confusion with family members and be sure to store them out of reach of children.

The laundry room. Eliminate harsh products and detergents with strong fragrances. When you see "fragrance" as an ingredient, know that's where many of the chemicals are hiding. Also, eliminate dryer sheets. They are chemical-laden and can cause allergic reactions. Even a simple Google search tells you that these simple products contain a fabric softener chemical and usually fragrance chemicals. Healthier products shouldn't contain any fragrances nor should the word "chemical" be in any description of something that touches clothing you wear on your body!

The garage. This is a biggie. My recommendation is to gather ALL the toxic chemicals in one big group—an organized group. Put like items together and eliminate expired or outdated products. Then based on what you're comfortable with and what you need right away, responsibly discard what you can. Put what you keep up on a shelf out of reach of children, or better yet, safely store items in a locked cabinet.

You can always take things a step further when it comes to making your home healthier. Change out air filters regularly, clean your washing machine, add LED bulbs, and clean the carpets using a non-toxic solution. There are endless ways to upgrade the health of your home, but eliminating the obvious toxins through responsibly discarding products containing chemicals is a good start.

• Creating Your Healthy Home •

It may feel overwhelming and almost impossible to make significant changes. There's a lot of information in this book and, as a coach, it would be irresponsible for me to tell you that you can make all of these changes right away. Remember, we talked about decision fatigue and indecision. My recommendation is to focus on one area at a time, which is why this book is broken into three sections: Creating a Healthy You, Creating a Healthy Kitchen, and Creating a Healthy Home. All of this depends upon how quickly you make decisions and how you adapt to change. The important thing is to go at your own pace and comfortability level, enlist support where you need it, and know that change takes time—so be patient with yourself in the process.

Here are some additional steps to create a healthier home. These are strategies that will help you eliminate any further excess and wake up to each day feeling like you're moving forward in a positive direction:

1. Stop shopping as a hobby. Find a free or low-cost activity instead. Sit outside, read a book, take a walk, or go see a movie. There are plenty of activities to do other than spend money on shopping. It's different if you actually need something like new towels or a lawn mower, but instead of shopping for random items or more clothing, put the money towards that dream vacation. It's that simple. Find an accountability partner you can call if you feel tempted. You owe it to yourself to create healthier habits.

2. Set up a donation station. Use four boxes labeled "Clothing," "Appliances/Technology," "Chemicals," and "Food Products." Start in the kitchen, set a timer for ten minutes and go through the pantry and cabinets, eliminating anything toxic. Do the same for each room. Once the boxes are full, get them in the car immediately and drop them off at the dump, a charity store such as Goodwill, or a food bank. But get rid of the stuff. Don't worry about selling or consigning. Just let it go, Elsa! The freedom you'll feel is worth any of the money you may recoup trying to sell these items. Continue this process until you have removed all unessential items. Once you feel like you've got things under control, add "Donate" boxes to each floor of your home so you can easily continue the process of decluttering on a regular basis.

3. Stop the junk mail and create a mail station. The only reason I go to the mailbox these days is to recycle. I live in a community where the mailboxes are in a centralized location, and the post office is allowed to junk up my box

with advertisements and flyers. I toss most of it in a big recycling bin next to the mailboxes before I even return home—what a waste of everyone's time and resources. If you're still receiving catalogs and mailers, go here: https://www.consumer.ftc.gov/articles/how-stop-junk-mail. If you're telling yourself you like to browse the catalogs, it may be time for a new hobby. This is unnecessary and is the gateway to purchasing, which is not the way to eliminate clutter and detox your home. Create ONE place in your home where the mail sits after you've gone to the mailbox and before you open it. When you open it, do it over a recycling bin. Toss all the advertisements, extra envelopes, etc. Flatten everything and put it in one of three folders: bills, action, or file.

4. Clean up before bed. This is a huge game changer. Take fifteen minutes to load the dishwasher, turn it on, wipe down countertops, prepare lunches for the following day. Waking up to a clean kitchen is a great way to start your day. Once you get into a groove, you will look forward to closing out the day this way because you know it makes for a better morning.

5. Create a capsule wardrobe. The 80/20 rule suggests we only wear twenty percent of the clothing we actually possess. Shop in your own closet and create a capsule wardrobe using a set number of pieces, then create outfits from those. Eliminating the eighty percent will simplify your decision-making each day and give you more space to see what you actually have on hand.

Whether you incorporate one or all of these steps, they will help you eliminate future clutter and create a healthier home. These strategies will also free you of some decision making, which then gives you time to do all the things you wished you had time for—or you can figure out ways to use this newly found time in your day.

• Exercise 1: Easy Tosses and Healthier Substitutions •

Over time, we may build up an intolerance to chemicals found within the home even though we could once withstand them. This happens for many reasons, including a combination of diet and medication, age, or simply an overabundance of chemicals that have accumulated in the home. Some of those intolerances can present themselves in the form of skin irritations, headaches, nasal issues, or fogginess. If you do suffer from allergies or simply want to detox your home, here are some easy tosses that may be adding to the clutter in your spaces and containing toxins. As you go through each section, check off what you eliminated.

LAUNDRY ROOM

❑ Bleach. Instead use baking soda, distilled white vinegar, and a natural stain remover.

❑ Febreze and other "scent-removers" and deodorizers only mask the odors. Deep clean where necessary.

❑ Dryer sheets. Replace with essential oil on a washcloth and toss it in for freshness. Use dryer balls or bypass the dryer and hang clothing made of synthetics.

BATHROOM

❑ Perfumes. Check the ingredients, even it means doing a Google search. You'd be surprised to discover what's in them.

❑ Facial cleansers. Choose fragrance-free products, and read the ingredients label.

❑ Shampoos/conditioners. Decide how many bottles you really need to have in the shower at one time.

❑ Anything containing "fragrances" on the ingredients label.

❑ Anything in an aerosol can. By default, you will reduce your carbon footprint and help the environment.

KITCHEN

❑ PAM cooking spray and similar products. Replace with olive oil or something similar.

❑ Anything in an aerosol can.

❑ Household cleaners with strong fragrances.

❑ Household cleaners with unidentifiable chemicals on the ingredients label.

Now let's learn how to choose better products and maintain a toxin-free home:

1. Read the ingredients label.
2. Use healthier versions. Baking soda makes a great cleaner for the bathtub. Add vinegar and some essential oils for a natural, clean concoction.
3. Eliminate duplicates. Set up an online account that allows you to repeat-order what you need when you're running low so you aren't using valuable real estate to house supplies.

Make better choices once you receive new information.

Now that you have new information, you're ready to replace the toxic items with a healthier version. Tackle these by category and check them off once you're finished:

- ❏ Cleaning products
- ❏ Laundry detergents
- ❏ Cosmetics

Go through each area of the home and centralize cleaning products using a cleaning caddy to make cleaning fast and simple. Here's where you want to place those caddies:

- ❏ Laundry room
- ❏ Under the kitchen sink
- ❏ Under the bathroom sinks

• Mindless vs. Mindful •

Mindless: Putting toxic products in and on our bodies then being surprised when we feel foggy or experience skin irritations.

Mindful: Replacing products with toxin- and fragrance-free ones that we can feel confident are positively contributing to our goals of a healthier lifestyle.

CHAPTER 9

Get Your Home In Order and Feel Great

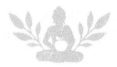

PHYSICAL CLUTTER IS A representation of what's happening in the mind.

By 2002, I'd been married for eight years and had two children. We had moved four times and were about to make a fifth move to be closer to the school we chose for our children. By this time, I was largely ruled by stuff and incredibly overwhelmed.

Not everyone gets into this predicament, but this is a problem in our modern world more and more. We have easy access to credit—more than anyone should have a right to—and access to stores around the clock through the internet. We want to reduce stress, and we're tempted by the promise that stuff will fix our lives and make our situation better.

I used to shop for the sake of shopping. Each trip to the store was essentially to fill myself up by purchasing items I did not need, hardly wanted, and rarely loved. I was subconsciously reacting to what my emotions and the media were telling all of us to do—buy, buy, buy. Don't think; just buy. Because I was in full-force motherhood mode, it also didn't occur to me to maybe engage in a hobby or activity that wouldn't include acquiring more things. Therefore, a time came when there wasn't one room in my home where I felt I could relax. Even the hidden clutter was calling to me in the form of unfiled paperwork, accumulated memorabilia, and clothing I had no intention of wearing. But for some reason, I continued to hang onto these things.

My thinking finally changed when I realized I'd bought a bigger house just to hold all of our stuff that we had accumulated. I was paying good money for real estate to store objects, most of which I didn't even like, thinking this is just how it was. I reached a point where I became so overwhelmed that I just wanted it to disappear. A bit extreme, but that was my reality. As I became more and more frustrated with the management of these things, one day I began pushing it out the door and into the garage. All of it—well, not quite. Out went the knick-knacks I never liked. Out went the boxes of *Metropolitan Home* magazines from the 1980s (that was tough purge). Out went the college textbooks on subjects that didn't interest me anymore. Out went the boxes of home accessories I was never going to use. Out went the old and ragged bath towels that weren't even worthy to use as rags. Out went the hand-me-down blender I never used. All of it out!

After almost filling a two-car garage, it became apparent that I had accumulated, among other things, three woks, eight pairs of gardening gloves, five one-gallon jugs of distilled water, eleven cookie sheets, five pairs of slippers, and three copies of the *American Heritage Dictionary*. Now it was time to make some decisions.

In order for me to organize and redecorate my home, I first needed to know how I wanted my home to feel. When I walked into a room, I wanted it to embrace me with a warm welcome—not attack me with visual distractions. I also wanted to know exactly where I could find something. I no longer wanted to spend time looking for a screwdriver when I needed it or endlessly search for my keys because I never put them in the same place when I walked in the door.

What I needed was a clear goal and a plan for organizing my spaces. With pen and paper in hand, I began to play around with furniture placement ideas on paper. I drew a rudimentary schematic of the space—not to scale—and sketched in the pieces of furniture. The plan included creating zones and designating space for various activities. I decided to place my books in one location, knowing exactly where to find them, and created a craft area to house all of those supplies. Once I was happy with the solution on paper, I began moving furniture. Then I could put our stuff away.

Before purging items, it was important to know I had the support of my family. I informed them of my intention to declutter and put aside items I thought they might want to have. As I began to donate things, I felt relieved and physically lighter. I continued asking myself: should it stay or should it go? The purging process continued. I kept the best and heaved the rest. I was on a first-name basis with the folks at Goodwill before too long.

Finally, I no longer had to search my house high and low for a particular book because I had all the books in one place. I no longer wondered where my keys were because they had a permanent home in the kitchen drawer where I placed them as soon as I entered the house. What a relief. Best of all, I wasn't constantly under pressure to do something about the clutter—it was gone! Purging what I no longer wanted or needed empowered me to take charge of my spaces. For once, I felt like I had created a cocoon for our family—a sacred place where we could retreat from the world's chaos into our own sanctuary.

At this point, I realized I needed to address two additional issues: time and systems. Now that I wasn't paralyzed by clutter, I had time to pursue interests I had been putting off. To make the most of my time, I created a priority list and scheduled time to do those activities. Further, I put systems in place to handle routine tasks such as mail, laundry, and family communications. These systems allowed me to quickly accomplish those tasks so I would not dread them but accomplish them and move on to other things.

The conscious path I took to create a small piece of heaven for myself was applicable to not only myself, but to many others. I had developed an easy-to-understand system that could help others create their own sanctuary from the outside world.

• Clutter: What Is It, Really?! •

Clutter is defined as "a collection of things lying about in an untidy mass." I like that definition. It's descriptive and you can easily picture what clutter is. And, if we look at the definition of *organizing*—to arrange things (likely clutter) in a structured order—we can actually organize clutter or things as opposed to *cleaning*—act of making something free of dirt, like dishes or clothing, for example.

I'd like to add a secondary definition for clutter I created during more than ten years spent organizing people's homes and commercial spaces:

Clutter = **indecision** + other people's expectations

People's expectations of us can include a family member asking us (or maybe guilting us) into taking a "treasured family heirloom," even when we don't have a place to put it. Now we're responsible for caring for this item, yet every time we look at it, we're reminded that we made a decision to do something for someone else even if we really didn't want to.

Indecision is the inability to make a quick decision, and sometimes we back off and don't make one at all. Then we remain stuck, unable to move forward.

The average person today has more stuff than is needed and, sadly, many people's credit card balances reflect this fact. Once, I heard someone say that if you want to know what you value you in your life, look at your credit and debit card statements—those will tell you because it's all the things you buy.

Clutter comes in many forms:

Physical. Too much stuff in your home space.

Mental. An overabundance of thoughts and mental chatter that goes unaddressed.

Spiritual or religious. Thoughts and perhaps doubts about one's beliefs.

Abundance clutter. The ability to buy without giving conscious thought to whether we're buying what we need or buying too much.

Calendar clutter. Putting too many commitments on our schedule that has us running around town and not entirely present at any one appointment or event.

Financial clutter. Unresolved debt, such as too many credit cards, failing to track expenses, and lack of budgeting or consideration for long-term savings.

Emotional Clutter. Unresolved issues from childhood, fractured relationships that haven't been worked through, or constant fear induced by anxiety issues.

"Sale" clutter. Stuff we purchased only because it's a two-for-one sale. Remember that it costs you nothing if you don't buy it.

• How Clutter Accumulates •

Beyond accumulating items through purchasing or accepting from others, indecision is the main reason we accumulate clutter. For example, when stuff accumulates on the kitchen counter, instead of deciding about where to put, it remains in a pile. And more and more accumulates. This happens for two reasons: either the items don't have a home or there's no system in place for transporting it to another room in the house where it actually lives.

Then the clutter gets ignored. When family members ask us about it, we brush it off, but subconsciously the accumulated clutter weighs on us.

Clutter also accumulates in the form of saying "yes" when we really needed to say "no" because we were already committed to do something else—this is calendar clutter. We need to understand what we're saying yes to. If the commitment requires resources we don't have—and I mean time or money OR the emotional capacity or energy—then we do things like avoid phone calls, don't show up, or forget to RSVP. This can make us look flaky, irresponsible, or like we just don't care.

It may get to a point where we are embarrassed and can't even admit to ourselves or others we need to shut down and reboot like a computer with a full memory or an overheated car.

The reality is that developing the habit of saying "let me think about it" instead of an immediate "yes," or just a "no, thank you" can help us avoid having to "fix" things later on. When people have expectations of us and we do not have sufficient boundaries in place or have a difficult time saying, "no, thank you," we can wind up taking on clutter such as an unnecessary coffee meeting, family furniture, or heading up the bake sale. These are just a few examples of clutter in the form of time, space, and resources.

And there's also mental clutter that surfaces when we are carrying around unresolved feelings about an issue with a family member or a friend. Maybe we keep repeating a conversation in our head that we'd like to have with this person, but we're afraid to. That mental clutter also needs decluttering. So whether you write a letter that you never send or you actually call the person who you have a grievance with, or talk with a close friend, or therapist, it's important to gain peace and clarity.

• The High Cost of Clutter •

Clutter not only costs money but also precious time and resources. Managing clutter can be a full-time job. It robs us of energy and the ability to sit and fully relax in our home. If we know we have a closet full of stuff demanding attention but we're ignoring it, our subconscious knows. And we'll never fully relax in our space.

Some people deal with clutter by avoiding it, which could come in the form of not spending much time at home. With all the daily demands, it's critical to have a place where we can relax and breathe easy at the end of the day.

Let's look at the effects of clutter on particular areas of our lives:

- Money. Many people spend good money on real estate to store their stuff, including items that could be sorted, downsized, or sold. The storage industry is estimated at $60 billion per year. People put things in storage with good intentions and either don't retrieve items or forget about them and wind up with a monthly payment for items they no longer even think about. You'll learn more about the cost of clutter in the What's it Worth exercise at the end of the chapter.

- Extra cleanup. When it's time to clean, clutter gets in the way. Avoid using countertops for storage. Instead, have a place for everything and put things away.

- Drains energy. Just looking at clutter can affect one's mood. Worse, when clutter accumulates and we think we're ignoring it, it still registers with our subconscious.

- Stops progress. Unrepaired items or incomplete tasks are a constant reminder of what one should have done and what one hasn't accomplished.

- Confuses the mind. Generally, clutter decreases one's focus and creates distractions that can easily throw one off balance.

• Eliminating Excess •

Purging, or editing as some call it, on a regular basis is important and necessary. Of course, if you decrease buying and edit regularly, you will reach a point where this task may be more seasonal or annual. Always keep in mind the 80/20 rule discussed earlier. Eliminating the 80% is a process, if that's what you decide is important to do.

Our first step, which we'll do in an exercise at the end of this chapter, is a brief room-by-room assessment. You'll want to go room by room and remove anything not relevant to the activity of that room. For example, the family room doesn't need to contain outdoor sporting equipment or makeup or plates and dishes, etc. The pantry does not need to contain collections of unrelated kitchen items or spare toilet paper.

Minimalism isn't a new concept, but a return to simpler times. Prior to consumerism taking over in the 1980s, people WERE actually living in a minimalistic way. If you look at the current decorating and design trends, they are very similar to the 1950s, when things were simpler. I'm not encouraging everyone to become minimalists but rather to think about things in a different way.

Today, people recognize that a simpler way of living can reduce stress by eliminating the overhead that includes a hefty mortgage, credit card bills, membership fees, and more. These are all things people have accepted as today's norm, but have our stress levels out of control.

Eliminating the excess comes in the form of reducing the trips to Target and shifting the hobby of shopping to walking in the park, for example. Shopping as a hobby only adds to our physical surroundings and potentially financial clutter. That money may better serve us in a savings account or a vacation fund.

Replacing the shopping hobby with exercise, fresh air, coffee with a friend, or something that will feed your soul and not deplete your bank account is a better option for maintaining calm in your mind, body and home.

Here are some easy tosses to launch your purge:

- Outdated and expired food products.
- Outdated technology. In the end, it costs more to hang on to it, and you'll feel relieved and lighter once it's gone.
- Old papers. Check with your accountant on how long you need to keep certain papers. Most documents can be scanned and placed on a hard drive and the physical documents can be shredded. Put all your important papers in one place (passports, marriage license, birth certificates, etc.)—a fireproof safe is handy for these items.
- Torn clothing, unless you're willing to repair it, but do it! Give yourself a deadline and if you don't meet it, get rid of it.
- Broken items. Same as torn clothing.
- Dead plants, unless you're willing to spend the time on bringing them back to life. But there's likely a good reason they're dead. Perhaps consider just one or two that you can make time to give love and attention to on a regular basis—and ones that don't require much watering.

Out of sight, out of mind – and this doesn't mean "hide" things in a closet, attic or storage unit. I promise you'll feel lighter! Focus on making the future simpler, more efficient, and full of joy instead the worrying about managing a bunch of physical things. Instead, go enjoy life's wonders.

• Put Yourself in the Driver's Seat •

When you're organizing categories such as crafts, collectibles, or hobby paraphernalia, ask yourself, "How much real estate do I want to give these items?" And instead of taking a passive role in this line of questioning and saying to yourself, "I don't have enough room for all this stuff," try reframing the language and instead say: "I'm going to allow half of my guest room closet to hold my craft supplies. Since I'm only allowing my crafts to take up this much space, I need to decide. I either take space from another category or I pare down what I currently have to fit that real estate."

Changing your perspective and the language you use will help you get the results you seek because you are empowered—you are no longer ruled by what you own. You become the ruler and have the last word!

• Cleaning vs. Organizing •

It's important to distinguish between cleaning and organizing. I already did this, but I'm going to define these terms again in case you immediately jumped to this chapter.

I hear people describe how they've been "cleaning" all day when really, they've been organizing. And when things are decluttered and organized, cleaning is a breeze!

Cleaning is the act of making something free of dirt, marks, or mess, especially by washing, wiping, or brushing. *Organizing* is the act of arranging things into a structured order OR into a structured or whole.

So you can see why when someone says they are going to clean their house, for example, oftentimes if you watch what they are doing or see the results, they've actually been organizing.

The goal for all of us is to eliminate the amount of time spent on household chores, or cleaning, so we can spend more time with our family, friends, and loved ones creating memories and enjoying life. Or you could simply spend time relaxing.

• Compartmentalize Your Cleaning •

If you're like most busy families today, finding a block of time to clean the entire house is nearly impossible and it may not go on the priority list at all, or you attempt to spot clean and it doesn't happen. Therefore, plan to compartmentalize your cleaning. For example, on Mondays, clean the upstairs bathrooms and the kitchen. On Tuesdays, clean the family room, and on Wednesday, plan to change and wash the sheets.

There's also the act of delegating and having family members help. Kids who learn these basic chores as part of growing up function more effectively as adults because they understand how to care for their surroundings. I can attest to this. I had my kids doing simple chores when they were as young as five, then gradually added more responsibility as they grew older and could handle more. As mentioned in Chapter 2, by teaching children valuable life skills, they will become independent adults.

So, get your family members involved!

• Exercise 1: The High-Cost of Clutter: Putting a Price Tag on Your Clutter •

This exercise is designed to help you to identify how much your clutter costs you based on the amount of space it's taking up in your home, storage unit or both.

•What's It Worth? •

When it comes to organizing, the goal is to know what you have and where it is. And there's more to it than having a place for everything.

It's important to give thought to how much space you're giving to a particular category/item. Most people take a passive stance on managing their belongings. They look at what they have and put it somewhere, rather than deciding how much space to allow for a specific category/function . Keep in mind that setting space limits may require downsizing what you have in a particular category—for example, collectibles, arts and crafts materials, gardening equipment, clothing, kitchen items, and so on. However, determining how much space you will give to a particular category/function, will give you more control over your stuff.

No matter where you live, you only have a finite amount of space. So, unless you're planning to move to a larger home, it's important to assess the existing space and how you're using it to ensure you're getting the most from your real estate investment. In some instances, I've coached individuals to pretend they're moving and see what they're willing to spend the time, money, and effort to move versus eliminating it in their existing space. Ask yourself whether you imagine particular items in your "new space." This will help you create a fresh space in your existing home.

• If You Own a Home •

Do the math and figure out how much your home's square footage is worth (dividing the purchase price of your home by its square footage). For a home, the value might be something like $125 per square foot, or as high as $250 to $500 per square foot if you live in California or a major city like New York or Chicago.

To figure out the value of a specific space, simply take its measurements. If your room is ten feet long and ten feet wide, that's a hundred square feet. Therefore, the value of the space in that room, based on $125 per square foot, is $12,500 of your overall investment.

If the room is completely cluttered, $12,500 of your overall real estate investment may be unusable. Look at the closets. The average size of a master bedroom walk-in closet is six feet long and six feet wide, or a total of forty-eight square feet. At $125 per square foot, that closet is worth $6,000. Do you currently have a closet jammed full of unused, unrecognizable items? You know, the closet you're afraid to go into?

The point being, many people invest in McMansions, thinking they need the extra space. In reality, many could actually live in smaller spaces if they considered the value of their things and how much space they want to give to those items.

Now you do the math.

Part One:

What is the value of your home $ _____
Divided by
Square footage = _____
Total $ _____ price per square foot

Part Two:

Size of the room: _____ total square footage (for example ten-by-ten feet = 100 square feet)
Multiplied by
Price per Square foot $_____
(take from Part One)
Equals
Total cost for housing your clutter $_____

• If You Rent Your Home •

You can also determine your real estate investment when you rent. If your rent is $1,200 per month for a 900-square-foot apartment, you're paying $1.33 per square foot, or $133.00 per month for room that's ten feet long and ten feet wide. If you have the room devoted to storage, ask yourself whether you'd be better off renting a storage facility for perhaps fifty dollars a month or reclaiming the space all together by decluttering and making it a functional space. Couples often wonder how they'll make space for a baby in a small city apartment, when the spare room is currently being used as an office or storage area.

So consider the money you're paying for the space and make some decisions.

Part One:

How much you pay per month for rent $_____

Divided by

Square footage = _____

Total $ _____ price per square foot

Part Two:

Size of the room: _____ total square footage
(for example ten-by-ten-feet = 100 square feet)

Multiplied by

Price per Square foot $_____
(take from Part One)

Equals

Total cost for housing your clutter $_____
per month

• Exercise 2: Compartmentalize Your Cleaning •

To make cleaning more efficient, in addition to a deep clean (scheduled as needed), consider compartmentalizing your cleaning to allow for freedom in your schedule so you're not having to spend all day Saturday or big chunks of time cleaning the house. Follow these simple tips:

Spot clean. Creating time in your schedule to clean for ten minutes to clean a (smaller) bathroom or fifteen minutes to wipe down the countertops in the kitchen and sweep the floor. Set up your "cleaning caddies" under each bathroom sink, the kitchen sink, and perhaps one in the laundry room/ closet, which would allow for quick and easy cleanups.

Make a schedule. Using the form below, create a schedule to organize the cleaning based on days of the week and time you have available. This is a great option too if you have children who can help with various chores as they reach certain ages. For example, kids as young as three and four could help with basic dusting, as long as you're not asking them to dust around fragile items. They can also help put their toys away. As children grow older, you can teach them to fold clothes or vacuum. Key is to lower your expectations as you "train" the little ones but stick to it and they can eventually take on more. Then when they go off to college, they can take care of themselves and their surroundings.

When Will I Clean?

	Sun	Mon	Tues	Wed	Thurs	Fri	Sat
Morning							
Mid-day							
Lunchtime							
Afternoon							
Early Evening							
Evening							

www.mindbodykitchenbook.com

1. **Determine number of areas you need to clean per week**—This would look something like this: Kitchen, Living Room, Dining Room, Bedrooms, Bathrooms.
2. **Breakdown each room with a list of tasks**—Using the Kitchen as an example, this would like: Wipe down countertops, Clean the floor (with the kitchen, we're assuming you're using the Clean out the Fridge method in Chapter 7 before you go grocery shopping).
3. **Consider the best time of days to accomplish these tasks**—Keep in mind that some tasks can only take 15 minutes. For example, cleaning the bathroom.
4. **Delegate**—Many tasks can be done by other members of the family, if that's your scenario. Consider "training" and assigning these exercises to other members of the family.
5. **Plan**—Enter the task in the allotted time slots.

Take 20. Work in twenty minutes at the end of the day to close up for the night. And, if you're attempting to eat healthier, close the kitchen before 8 p.m. by loading and running the dishwasher, then put away any hand-washed dishes, wipe down countertops and take out the trash. Then turn off the lights and leave the room. Find another activity after 8 p.m. to keep you occupied and out of the kitchen for those last-minute snacks.

What are three ways you can rethink your cleaning routine to maximize your time and delegate responsibility, freeing you up to get in some exercise and movement or meal prep for the week?

1. _____

2. _____

3. _____

Returning to the ideas in Chapter 8: "Detox Your Home," in what ways could you improve the quality of cleaning products you're using, both for surfaces and skin?

_____

_____

_____

• Mindless vs. Mindful •

Mindless: Bringing more new items into the home without eliminating equal number of items to avoid more and more clutter.

Mindful: A clear plan to eliminate the unnecessary items no longer relevant to your life today.

Putting it All Together

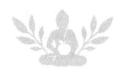

CONGRATULATIONS, YOU'VE MADE IT to the end of the book! Hopefully by now you've completed all the exercises at the end of each chapter and you've been making progress.

Your journey began with the importance of a solid foundation and how self-compassion is the key to long-lasting change. Taking care of yourself first, setting boundaries, and creating rituals to support yourself with love is critical in the process of creating a healthier lifestyle.

You also learned the basics of nutrition. This isn't a nutrition book and I'm not a nutritionist (I'm a certified health and wellness coach), although I did study more than a hundred different dietary theories while earning my certification. I have provided you with simple steps to understand the key pitfalls people make when they are trying to decide what to eat. If you follow the guidelines in this book, along with what's listed below, you're way ahead of most people:

1. Eat more plants. Green, leafy vegetables are underrated. They provide daily nutrients most people don't get on a regular basis. Yes, more nutrients than even protein.

2. Eat less or no meat. If you do eat meat, choose organic, antibiotic free so your body is also free of chemicals. You ingest what the animals ingested!

3. Read ingredients labels. ONLY choose packaged foods with five ingredients or less. You should know what the ingredients are without Googling them.

4. Drink more water. This is essential for a well-functioning body. Remember the car analogy. Water is like the oil. It's essential to a healthy, well-running body.

5. Less is more. Adopt this mantra and you'll not only minimize your portion sizes, but create simple surroundings.

6. Quality over quantity. Choosing quality ingredients and eating less processed foods will have you on the road to a healthier lifestyle.

7. Move. Exercise and movement are necessary. However you get it, get it! Take the stairs, park farther away, go to the gym, stretch at home, have a dance party. Do whatever it takes to get moving on a regular basis.

8. Create a healthy kitchen. Using the simple strategies and techniques provided in this chapter, you will create simple, healthy meals in your kitchen on a regular basis. Get in there, experiment, practice, get dirty, and strengthen that muscle.

9. Create an organized kitchen. An organized kitchen will have you functioning at top speed. Eliminate distractions, act like a restaurant, clean up afterwards (empty sink before closing time), and then get out of Dodge once you're done.

10. Plan, plan, and plan! A well-executed event only happens after a solid plan is put into place. Taking time on the

weekend (or "your weekend") to plan and prep for the week will save you time and have you eating healthier all week long.

11. Detox your home. Rid yourself of products containing toxic chemicals, whether it's in the laundry room, under the kitchen sink, or in the medicine cabinet.

12. Declutter and organize. Create a sanctuary where you can breathe easy and relax, free of distractions. Understand how much clutter is costing you and how you can reclaim time and space to reduce stress and get the most out of life. You've only got one, so make the most of it—NOW!

Remember, if I can do it, so can you!

• Resources •

Downloadable exercises available here:
www.mindbodykitchenbook.com

Mind Body Kitchen Blog:
www.staceycrew.com/blog

Transform You & Your Kitchen online course:
www.staceycrew.com/mindbodykitchencourse

Apps

Meditation
    Calm
    Headspace
    Insight Timer
    Jason Stephenson on YouTube
    Michael Sealey on YouTube

Books

A Complaint Free World: How to Stop Complaining and Start Enjoying the Life You Always Wanted, by Will Bowen

Big Magic, by Elizabeth Gilbert

Crazy Sexy Diet: Eat Your Veggies, Ignite Your Spark, and Live Like You Mean It, by Kris Carr

Clear Your Clutter with Feng Shui: Free Yourself from Physical, Mental, Emotional, and Spiritual Clutter Forever by Karen Kingston

Everything is Figureoutable, by Marie Forleo

FOOD: What the Heck Should I Eat?, by Mark Hyman, M.D.

Intuitive Eating, A Revolutionary Anti-Diet Approach, by Evelyn Tribble, MS and Elyse Resch

Judgement Detox: Release the Beliefs That Hold You Back from Living a Better Life, by Gabrielle Bernstein

Mothering with Courage: The Mindful Approach to Becoming a Mom Who Listens More, Worries Less, and Loves Deeply, by Bonnie Compton, APRN, BC, CPNP

Non-Toxic: Guide to Living Healthy in a Chemical World by Aly Cohen, M.D. and Frederick S. vom Saal, Ph.D.

Safe People: How to Find Relationships That Are Good For You and Avoid Those That Aren't by Dr. Henry Cloud & Dr. John Townsend

Self-Compassion: The Proven Power of Being Kind To Yourself, by Kristen Neff, Ph.D.

The Earth Diet: Your Complete Guide to Living Using Earth's Natural Ingredients by Liana Werner-Gray

The Detox Prescription: Supercharge Your Health, Strip Away Pounds, and Eliminate the Toxins Within by Woodson Merrell, M.D.

The Four Agreements: A Practical Guide to Personal Freedom by Don Miguel Ruiz

The Gift of Change, by Mariann Williamson

The Gifts of Imperfection: Let Go of Who You Think You're Supposed to Be and Embrace Who You Are, by Brene Brown

The Juicing Bible, by Pat Crocker

The Power of Intention: Learning to Create Your World Your Way by Dr. Wayne Dyer

The Power of Now: A Guide to Spiritual Enlightment by Eckhart Tolle

The Real Food Grocery Guide, by Maria Marlowe

The Science of Skinny Cookbook, by Dee McCaffrey, CDC

Untamed, by Glennon Doyle

Women Code: Perfect Your Cycle, Amplify Your Fertility, Supercharge Your Sex Drive, and Become a Power Source, by Alisa Vitti, HHC & Founder of Flo Living

You Are a Badass, by Jen Sincero

You Can Heal Your Life, by Louise Hay

Documentaries

Fat, Sick and Nearly Dead
Fed Up
Forks Over Knives
Hungry for Change
In Defense of Food
Minimalism
What the Health

Podcasts

Dear Gabby: Become the Happiest Person You Know with Gabby Bernstein

Good Life Project with Jonathan Fields

On Purpose with Jay Shetty

The Goop Podcast

The Minimalists with Joshua Fields Millburn & Ryan Nicodemus

The Smart Human with Dr. Aly Cohen

Unlocking Us with Brene Brown

We Can Do Hard Things with Glennon Doyle

Online Grocery

Amazon Prime
Brandless.com
Thrivemarket.com
Vitacost.com

Clutter Reduction

The Life-Changing Magic of Tidying Up: The Japanese Art of Decluttering and Organizing by Marie Kondo

Seven Steps to Unclutter Your Life by Donna Smallin

www.theminimalists.com

• Additional Home Systems •

FAMILY COMMUNICATIONS CENTER

Even in a technologically-advanced world, we can't always avoid paper, especially if we have school-aged kids. Keeping a family calendar that everyone can see in a prominent location can help everyone juggle activities and commitments.

The Family Communications Center (FCC) is your mission control, where everyone can see the family calendar of activities and events. It's also where you may want to place paperwork (in a binder) such as phone lists, business cards, takeout menus, a running lists of household projects, and baby items needed/wanted. Don't overload this section with old information. You want it active and current!

Carve out a zone for the FCC on the inside of the pantry door or on a wall in the mudroom or laundry room, whatever is central and convenient to where you spend the majority of your time in the home. Maintain control of the family schedule and activities by including the following in your FCC area:

- Bulletin board/chalkboard. Hang shopping lists, an envelope for invitations/activities, phone numbers, hot lunch menu, etc. Be choosey about what you add to the board and routinely purge.
- Pens/pencils. Use colored pencils to indicate different categories (for example, purple for kids, green for work

activities, red for social activities).
- Calendar. A two- to three-month calendar is a great way to see what's current and what's on the horizon.
- Three to four envelopes or containers. Label envelopes "invites," "coupons," and "bills to pay," and any other categories relevant to you for important papers.

Establish a place in the FCC to place a three-ring binder that can house information you refer to on a regular basis. Here are possible sections:

- Phone list
- Business card holder sheets
- Household projects to complete (keep a list and priortize)
- Takeout menus

You can easily customize your Family Communication Center

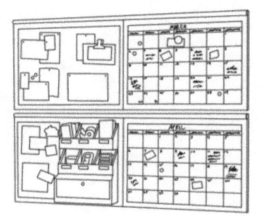

• Mail Center •

Mail becomes an issue when there's no system in place for it. For example, if you have no "landing" place, it can wind up in different places throughout the house, or you're not sure what to do with it.

There are three choices when it comes to mail: file, act on it, or toss. An easy toss: solicitations you're not in the market for.

<u>WHAT YOU NEED</u>

- "Bills to be paid" container
- Trash can
- Envelopes, stamps, a pen, and note paper or stationery

<u>WHERE TO PUT IT</u>

In the front hall or near the family communications center. Avoid using a drawer or an out-of-sight container.

<u>SYSTEM</u>

So everyone's responsible for their own mail, designate an in-box for each member of the family. Open your mail with the trashcan handy. Immediately toss any unsolicited direct mail offers unless you've decided previously it's something you've been searching for. Throw away the envelopes the mail arrives in and place the bills in "bills to be paid" container to avoid misplacing them. Put anything to be filed directly in a reference file cabinet in your office.

• Recipes •

You can easily organize recipes in three ways.

<u>WHAT YOU NEED</u>

- A traditional recipe box. Some find this to be a way to stay connected to memories from times when they were younger.
- A binder with clear sheet protectors. This keeps the recipe clean and maintains organization so you can easily find what you're looking for.
- On Pinterest. This is a physically clutter-free option allowing for easy access anywhere.

Remember, you can access many recipes online, so be particular about which recipes you choose to keep a hard copy of in your physical space. Of course, Mom's apple pie recipe that she originally wrote on an index card deserves a special place, in a special box in your kitchen! If you're using a recipe box or binder, label the sections as follows:

- Breakfast/Lunch
- Dinner/Appetizers
- Casseroles/Soups/Stews
- Desserts/Vegetable Dishes
- Snacks/Other (you choose!)

WHERE TO PUT IT

Place the loose recipe binder or the recipe box in the kitchen where it is handy—near the cookbooks. If you choose to keep your recipes on your computer, there are many electronic solutions on the market today. Do a Google search for "recipe software" to locate a vendor.

• Beverage Station •

WHAT YOU NEED

Glasses, cups, spoons (if you're making coffee/tea/hot chocolate), coffee/tea (if you're making this), coffee grinder, tea infuser, etc.

WHERE TO PUT IT

Locate near the fridge and/or sink (or near to the serving zone so you already have some items available to you. For example, cups and spoons.)

Tips: House items in a cabinet or basket. Try not to clutter the counter with all of these items for the drink station, although you could use a tray to create a usable display for these items.

• Three-Day Jumpstart •

Preparation Guide

Welcome to the **Three-Day Clean Eating Jumpstart**. I've got you covered on what you need to do one week prior to the challenge, two days before and one day before you begin. If you follow this guide and the subsequent meal plan, in just three days you will kick sugar, reduce cravings and inflammation in the body, and gain more energy!

It's best to start on a Monday so you can prepare the weekend before; there are still some things you want to accomplish before then.

ONE WEEK BEFORE

Having support in anything we do is important to achieving success! That includes the people closest to us. I suggest talking with your friends and family beforehand so they can provide you with support. Better yet, get your whole family on board for the three days. To create a solid foundation for the upcoming challenge, discuss how you feel and communicate this to the supportive people in your life. Talk about your intentions and your goal(s). And, again, see if anyone wants to join you in your clean eating adventure!

It's important to identify a *why*, especially when you're in the middle of the challenge and you're questioning, "WHY did I decide to do this?" "WHAT was I thinking?!" So, take a few minutes to identify and write three specific reasons WHY you are doing the challenge so you can keep these in mind throughout the three-day process.

1.

2.

3.

I also suggest journaling or freewriting about your whys. For example, maybe you want to detox your body. Use freewriting to elaborate on that statement. Describe how you want your body to eliminate fatigue and bloating. Or perhaps you want to fit into the jeans that have been hanging in your closet for six months. Maybe you have a specific weight loss goal in mind, so express the feelings surrounding that why. Whatever it is, remember that food is sometimes the symptom to the underlying issues and ultimately addressing those issues will allow you to clean up your act for good. Whatever it is, you will learn to eat cleaner and ultimately feel better!

TWO DAYS BEFORE

- Organize your fridge. Clear a specific spot in the fridge for the food you will eat during the jumpstart. Better yet, clear the clutter and stock up on clean food so you can continue once you've completed the challenge. Read the following blog post to guide to easily organizing your fridge: https://staceycrew.com/organized-kitchen/

- Shop for groceries using the shopping list below.

ONE DAY BEFORE

- Remind your family and friends about the week ahead and ask them for their continued support.

- Organize your food. For example, snacks can be packed up for the three days in small storage containers.

- Pack your lunch bag. If you'll be taking your food on-the-go (whether to work or a meeting) have it ready to grab and go in the morning after you've had your Day 1 Breakfast. On Monday evening, pack your Tuesday lunch and on Tuesday night pack for Wednesday.

Hints

Ask yourself what you can prepare today so you don't have to make a full-blown meal each night of the week. Portion my snacks for the week so you're not scrambling, or worse, getting a candy bar from the vending machine at work.

If you have a scale, weigh yourself. Remember, the clean-eating challenge isn't designed for you to lose weight, but for you to reduce sugar and have more energy. For some, the number is important, so I won't discourage a weigh in. However, I do encourage you to become aware of how you feel before you begin the challenge, how you feel during, and how you feel afterwards.

Now you have the tools!

TIPS

Here are some food preparation tips for your Three-Day Jumpstart Meal Plan to help you meal plan efficiently. The tips are broken down by breakfast, lunch and dinner.

- **Breakfast**: On Monday morning, triple the recipe so you have enough for all three days. This will save time.

- **Lunch:** You can prepare the lunches in Mason jars (large sixteen ounces) or Tupperware-like storage containers for all three days because you will store a dressing separately so it won't wilt the romaine lettuce.

- **Dinner**: Simple recipes are provided so you can take your pick, but if you're pressed for time during the weeknights and you're considering the baked chicken option, think about cooking it on Sunday to heat up on Monday. You could do the same with the bean burgers. Also, there a couple recipes that call for quinoa, so you can easily prepare that and some steamed veggies on Sunday, too.

Now it's time to get moving. Get your support system in place, clean and organize your fridge, go shopping and meal prep!

For added support, you can join the Mind Body Kitchen Facebook group (www.facebook.com/groups/mindbodykitchen) and post questions and comments as you proceed through the Three-Day Clean Eating Jumpstart.

THREE-DAY JUMPSTART MEAL PLAN

	DAY ONE	DAY TWO	DAY THREE
First	Warm lemon water	Warm lemon water	Warm lemon water
Break-fast	**Choose two:** (a) avocado toast, (b) green smoothie, (c) hard-boiled egg, (d) oatmeal with maple syrup or (e) wildberry/banana smoothie.	**Choose two:** (a) avocado toast, (b) green smoothie, (c) hard-boiled egg, (d) oatmeal with maple syrup or (e) wildberry/banana smoothie.	**Choose two:** (a) avocado toast, (b) green smoothie, (c) hard-boiled egg, (d) oatmeal with maple syrup or (e) wildberry/banana smoothie.
Water	**Drink** at least 16 oz. of water this morning	**Drink** at least 16 oz. of water this morning	**Drink** at least 16 oz. of water this morning
Snack	**Choose two:** (a) apple, (b) carrots and hummus or (c) strawberries	**Choose two:** (a) apple, (b) carrots and hummus or (c) strawberries	**Choose two:** (a) apple, (b) carrots and hummus or (c) strawberries
Water	**Drink** at least 16 oz. of water this morning	**Drink** at least 16 oz. of water this morning	**Drink** at least 16 oz. of water this morning

Lunch	**Choose one:** (a) salad (with beans or a bean burger) or (b) veggie sandwich **AND** a piece of fruit (orange or apple)	**Choose one:** (a) salad (with chicken or salmon) or (b) veggie sandwich **AND** a piece of fruit (orange or apple)	**Choose one:** (a) salad (add chickpeas or navy beans) or (b) taco **AND** a piece of fruit (orange or apple)
Water	**Drink** at least 16 oz. of water this morning	**Drink** at least 16 oz. of water this morning	**Drink** at least 16 oz. of water this morning
Snack	**Choose two:** (a) kale chips, (b) raw chocolate balls or (c) strawberry-banana smoothie	**Choose two:** (a) kale chips, (b) raw chocolate balls or (c) strawberry-banana smoothie	**Choose two:** (a) kale chips, (b) raw chocolate balls or (c) strawberry-banana smoothie
Dinner	**Choose one:** (a) baked chicken, cauliflower and spinach or (b) Tacos with cauliflower or sauteed spinach	**Choose one:** (a) bean burgers, steamed broccoli and sweet potato or (b) tacos with steamed broccoli	**Choose one:** (a) baked chicken with sauteed spinach and sweet potato or (b) tacos with sauteed spinach
Water	**Drink** at least 16 oz. of water this morning	**Drink** at least 16 oz. of water this morning	**Drink** at least 16 oz. of water this morning
Snack	Apple or orange	Apple or orange	Apple or orange
Before Bed	Disconnect from social media at least 30 minutes before bed and read a book.	Take a warm Epsom salt bath to help detox your body. Drink a caffeine-free tea.	Listen to a sleep meditation as you fall asleep (search YouTube.com)
Sleep	Aim to get 8 hours of sleep.	Aim to get 8 hours of sleep.	Aim to get 8 hours of sleep.

SHOPPING LIST

Baking

- ❑ 1 small bag Almond Meal
- ❑ 1 small pkg. Cacao Powderw
- ❑ Unbleached all-purpose flour (Bean Burgers)

Breads/Grains

- ❑ Bread: Ezekiel or whole grain or whole wheat
- ❑ 1 pkg. tortilla wraps
- ❑ 3 cups oatmeal (preferably from bulk food section)
- ❑ 1 ½ cups quinoa (package okay or bulk section is usually less expensive)
- ❑ Sesame seeds (for spinach salad)

Canned

- ❑ 2 cans of organic black beans (one if you're not doing bean burgers)

Condiments

- ❑ 1 small bottle pure maple syrup
- ❑ Sea Salt (versus table salt-healthier!)
- ❑ 1 jar coconut oil
- ❑ Extra-virgin olive oil
- ❑ Balsamic vinegar
- ❑ Apple cider vinegar
- ❑ Honey (for Balsamic Apple Cider Vinegar dressing)
- ❑ Mustard
- ❑ Salsa
- ❑ 1 tub of hummus
- ❑ 1 container almond milk

Dairy

- ❑ 6 eggs (3 if you're not eating bean burgers)—organic and cage-free, if possible
- ❑ 1 pkg. Mexican cheese
- ❑ Sour cream (bean burgers and tacos)

Frozen section

- ❑ 6 cups of wild blueberries

Meat

- ☐ 1 small piece Salmon
- ☐ 1-3 Organic Chicken Breasts
- ☐ 1 lb. Ground Beef (organic, grass-fed)

Produce

- ☐ 2 medium-sized organic lemons
- ☐ 1 container of strawberries (large container for smoothie)
- ☐ 6 organic apples
- ☐ 2-3 oranges (if you're not eating apples or enjoy fruit and want to snack!)
- ☐ 5-6 bananas (adjust if you're not doing smoothies or only doing one)
- ☐ 6 nearly-ripened avocados (3 if you're not doing the avocado toast but you may want to add some to salad—you estimate based on how much you like avocados)

- ☐ 3-4 heads of Romaine lettuce
- ☐ 1 container of cherry tomatoes
- ☐ 2 large tomatoes (veggie sandwich and salad)
- ☐ 2 medium-sized cucumbers
- ☐ 1 package of baby organic carrots
- ☐ 1 head of broccoli
- ☐ 1 head of cauliflower
- ☐ 2-3 medium-sized sweet potatoes
- ☐ 2 yellow peppers (salad, bean burgers, tacos)
- ☐ 1 red pepper (bean burgers)
- ☐ 1 small white onion
- ☐ 1 bag spinach
- ☐ 1 bag kale
- ☐ Fresh garlic
- ☐ Fresh cilantro

• Simple Recipes•

First thing in the morning

LEMON WATER

Ingredients:
- ½ medium-sized fresh (preferably organic) lemon
- 6-8 oz. warm tap water

Directions:
1. Fill glass with 6-8 oz. of warm tap water.
2. Cut lemon in half and squeeze into warm water.
3. Drink up!

Breakfast Options

AVOCADO TOAST

Ingredients:
- One piece of whole-wheat or Ezekiel bread
- ½ ripened avocado

Directions:
4. Toast bread and spread ½ of avocado.
5. Add salt & pepper to taste.
6. For additional nutritional benefits, add sprouts and cucumber (thin slices).

GREEN SMOOTHIE

Ingredients:
- 1 cup spinach
- 1 cup kale
- ½ banana
- ½ cup of water

Directions:
- Put all in a blender and blend until mixture reaches a smooth consistency.

OATMEAL WITH MAPLE SYRUP

Ingredients:

- 1 cup oatmeal (use organic—this can be purchased from bulk section of Whole Foods or similar type store). To eat clean, do not purchase packaged oatmeal. These typically have inflammatory ingredients. Please read the label.
- 1 tablespoon of pure maple syrup.

Directions:

1. Bring 1 ½ cups of water to a boil.
2. Add oatmeal and stir and reduce heat to medium.
3. Cook for 4-5 minutes or until water is absorbed, stirring throughout.
4. Place in a bowl.
5. Add 1 tablespoon of maple syrup.

Note: If you plan to triple this recipe, follow steps one through three for three cups of oatmeal and store in sealed container in the refrigerator. When you're ready to reheat for days two and three, add 1 tablespoon of maple syrup before reheating for thirty seconds in the microwave.

....

BLUEBERRY SMOOTHIE

Ingredients:

- 2 cups frozen blueberries
- 1 banana
- 1 cup water (add other fruit and vegetables, if desired; a small handful of spinach or kale is a good add)

Directions:

1. Combine the wild blueberries, bananas, and water in the blender. Blend the ingredients until smooth and well combined. Serves 1-2 people.

Snack Options

CARROTS & HUMMUS

Ingredients:

- 6 baby organic carrots
- 1 tablespoon of hummus

Directions:

1. Enjoy!

KALE CHIPS

Ingredients:

- 2 cups kale (bagged kale is okay and easy)
- Olive oil
- Salt

Directions:

1. Preheat oven to 425 degrees.
2. Place kale on a baking sheet.
3. Lightly sprinkle with salt and olive oil.
4. Place in oven for 15-17 minutes or until crisp.
5. Place in a Tupperware-like container until ready to eat.

RAW CHOCOLATE BALLS
(The Earth Diet 10-minute Recipe Book)

Ingredients:

- 1 cup nut meal (Almond or Cashew)
- ¼ cup cacao powder
- 3 tablespoons pure maple syrup or raw honey (I prefer maple syrup; it's easier to work with and sweeter!)

Directions:

1. Mix the three ingredients together in a bowl. Keep mixing until the mixture becomes semi-solid.
2. Roll the mixture into ½-inch balls in size.

Notes: This makes 1 ½ cups, takes about 5 minutes, and serves 8, so you have enough to snack on for a few days.

Variations: If you're craving salty foods, add a ¼ teaspoon of sea salt to the mixture. You can also add a ¼ teaspoon of pure vanilla extract.

....

STRAWBERRY/BANANA SMOOTHIE

Ingredients:

- 1 banana
- 1 cup strawberries
- 1 cup almond milk

Directions:

1. Place ingredients in a blender or Magic Bullet.
2. Blend until mixture is smooth.

· ·

Lunch Options

· ·

QUINOA SALAD

Ingredients:

- 2 cups romaine lettuce
- ½ cup diced cherry tomato
- ½ cup cucumber
- ½ avocado
- ½ cup of quinoa
- Salt & pepper to taste (use organic sea salt)
- Dressing if desired (see recipes below)

Directions:

1. Use a 16 oz. mason jar or a storage container.
2. Add tomatoes first, then the romaine lettuce, cucumber and quinoa.
3. Cut the avocado fresh, if possible and add when you eat, along with the S&P and dressing (see below for dressing recipe).

Variation: Add Chicken, Salmon or a Bean Burger for added protein and flavor.

VEGGIE SANDWICH

Ingredients:

- Two slices of bread
- Romaine Lettuce
- Thin-sliced tomato
- Cucumber sliced thin
- ½ avocado
- Salt & pepper to taste

Directions:

- Assemble sandwich.

Note: If you're making the sandwich in the morning to take with you and you're planning on adding avocado, take ½ an avocado with you and slice and add when you're ready to eat.

Salad Dressings

BALSAMIC APPLE CIDER VINEGAR
(The Earth Diet 10-Minute Recipe book)

Ingredients:
- 1 tablespoon apple cider vinegar
- 1 tablespoon organic balsamic vinegar
- 1 teaspoon honey

Directions:

- Mix all ingredients together in a bowl until combined.

MUSTARD VINAIGRETTE
(The Earth Diet 10-Minute Recipe book)

Ingredients:

- ⅓ cup extra virgin olive oil
- 1 ½ teaspoons apple cider vinegar
- 1 teaspoon garlic, minced
- 1 tablespoon mustard
- 14 teaspoon black pepper
- ¼ teaspoon salt (sea salt)

Directions:

- Mix all ingredients into a bowl until well combined.

Dinner Options

BAKED CHICKEN

Ingredients:

- 1 piece of organic chicken
- Salt & pepper

Directions:

1. Carefully wash chicken, pat dry with a paper towel, and place on baking sheet.
2. Add salt & pepper.
3. Bake at 350 degrees for 30-35 minutes.

BAKED SALMON

Ingredients:
- 1 piece of salmon

Directions:

1. Place salmon on baking sheet.
2. Add salt & pepper.
3. Bake at 350 degrees for 13-15 minutes.

BEAN BURGERS

Ingredients:

- 1.5 cups black beans (one can), cooked (drain once cooked)
- 1 large yellow (and/or red) pepper, chop into small pieces
- 1 small white onion, diced
- 2 garlic cloves, crushed
- 1 large tomato, chopped into small pieces
- 3 tablespoons of fresh chopped cilantro)
- ½ cup all-purpose unbleached flour
- 2 eggs, room temperature
- Sea salt and black pepper

Directions:

1. Preheat oven to 375 degrees.
2. Combine all ingredients in a large bowl, stir well to combine (add more flour if not binding).
3. Season with the sea salt and black pepper.
4. Make hamburger-size patties, placing them on a lightly greased baking sheet (use coconut oil).
5. Pop in the oven for about 18-20 minutes (longer, if needed).

Condiments: If you want to use ketchup on your bean burger, use organic and use only 1 tablespoon.

STEAMED BROCCOLI

Ingredients:

- 1 head of fresh broccoli
- Salt & pepper

Directions:

1. Wash broccoli and pat dry.
2. Cut the crowns of the broccoli from the stem into bite-sized pieces.
3. Put 1-inch of water into a saucepan and bring to a boil.
4. Place the broccoli into the boiling water, reduce the heat to medium, cover, and allow it to cook for about 5 minutes (make sure you can pierce it before straining).
5. Strain in a colander.
6. Serve with salt & pepper (no butter for clean eating).

STEAMED CAULIFLOWER

Ingredients:

- 1 head of fresh cauliflower
- Salt & pepper

Directions:

1. Wash cauliflower and pat dry.
2. Cut the crowns of the cauliflower from the stem into bite-sized pieces.
3. Put 1-inch of water into a saucepan and bring to a boil.
4. Place the cauliflower into the boiling water, reduce the heat to medium, cover, and allow it to cook for about 5 minutes (make sure you can pierce it before straining).

5. Strain in a colander.
6. Serve with salt and pepper (no butter for clean eating).

SAUTEED SPINACH

Ingredients:

- 2 cups fresh spinach
- Salt & pepper
- Olive oil

Directions:

1. Wash and pat dry spinach.
2. Heat sauté pan on medium-high.
3. Add olive oil and allow to warm for 30 seconds.
4. Add spinach and sauté.
5. Add salt & pepper to taste.

SWEET POTATO FRIES

Ingredients:

- 2 medium-sized sweet potatoes
- Coconut oil
- Salt & pepper

Directions:

1. Wash sweet potatoes. Not necessary to peel.
2. Dice into thin, French fry size pieces.
3. Place on lightly greased baking sheet (use coconut oil).
4. Add salt and pepper.

5. Bake at 350 degrees for 18-20 minute (longer, if needed, for crispier fries).

· ·

SPINACH SALAD

Ingredients:

- 2 cups of fresh spinach
- ½ cucumber diced
- Sesame seeds
- Dressing

Directions:

1. Wash and pat the spinach dry.
2. Place in a large bowl.
3. Dice cucumber and add to spinach.
4. Sprinkle with sesame seeds.
5. Add dressing.

· ·

TACOS
(The Earth Diet 10-Minute Recipe book)

Ingredients:

- With meat (1 pound organic, grass-fed beef)
- Whole-wheat tortilla wraps
- Romaine lettuce
- Diced yellow pepper
- Black beans (canned works well)
- Salsa

- Organic Mexican cheese (to keep it really clean, eliminate the cheese)
- Sour cream (sparingly)
- Fresh cilantro
- Salt & pepper to taste

For seasoning:

- 1 teaspoon turmeric
- 1 teaspoon cumin
- 1 teaspoon onion powder
- ½ teaspoon paprika
- Dash of cayenne pepper

*For a quicker meal, use a pre-packaged taco seasoning.

Directions:

1. Heat a large frying pan with olive oil, then add the beef and spices. Use a wooden spoon to break up the beef and combine the mixture well. Cook for approximately 8-10 minutes on medium-high heat.
2. Lightly brown tortillas in pan using a little olive oil.
3. Assemble tacos to your liking.

CPSIA information can be obtained
at www.ICGtesting.com
Printed in the USA
BVHW030913221121
622224BV00001B/34